GOOD MOURN-ING

GOOD MOURN-ING

HONEST CONVERSATIONS ABOUT GRIEF AND LOSS

Sally Douglas and Imogen Carn

murdoch books

Sydney | London

Published in 2023 by Murdoch Books, an imprint of Allen & Unwin

Murdoch Books Australia
Cammeraygal Country
83 Alexander Street, Crows Nest NSW 2065
Phone: +61 (0)2 8425 0100
murdochbooks.com.au
info@murdochbooks.com.au

Murdoch Books UK
Ormond House, 26–27 Boswell Street, London WC1N 3JZ
Phone: +44 (0) 20 8785 5995
murdochbooks.co.uk
info@murdochbooks.co.uk

A catalogue record for this book is available from the National Library of Australia

A catalogue record for this book is available from the British Library

ISBN 978 1 92261 631 9 Australia

Cover and text design by Madeleine Kane
Cover and internal illustrations by Sarah Campbell/The Illustration Room

Typeset by Madeleine Kane
Printed and bound by CPI Group (UK) Ltd, Croydon CR0 4YY

We acknowledge that we meet and work on the traditional lands of the Cammeraygal people of the Eora Nation and pay our respects to their elders past, present and future.

10 9 8 7 6 5 4 3

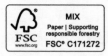

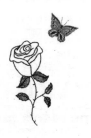

For our mums, Rose and Vanessa, and for
all those missing someone they love.

This book is for you.

CONTENTS

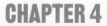

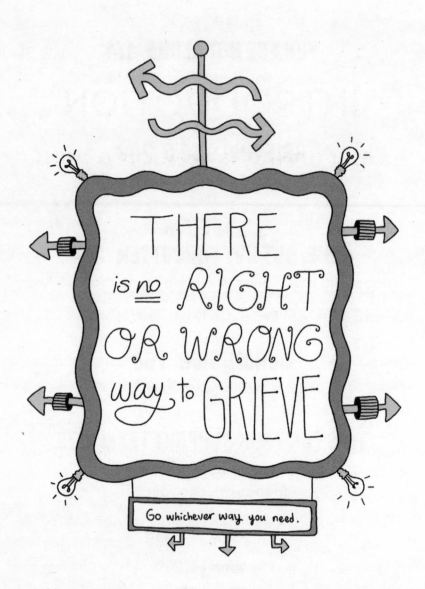

INTRODUCTION
Ugly crying is welcome here

Loss is a natural part of life. It's something that we will all inevitably experience, yet we don't know how to talk about it. When someone in your life dies, everything around you feels alien. Nothing makes sense anymore. You can try to imagine grief or prepare yourself for it, but until death comes knocking on the door of someone you love, it's hard to grasp the magnitude of it.

If you've picked up this book, you're probably in a painful place and trying to survive what feels completely unsurvivable. We get it. Grief is a wild ride – it's lonely, confusing and can feel like your world has been turned inside out and upside down. Because, frankly, it has!

We're Sally and Imogen (aka Sal and Im), hosts of the Good Mourning podcast. We became fully-fledged grievers when our mums died suddenly, only months apart. Like you, we know firsthand how tremendously difficult, earth-shattering and life-changing grief can be.

Maybe you're a long-time listener of our podcast (if so, hello). Or perhaps you've never heard of us but have picked up this book because you're deep in grief and desperately need some extra support. Whatever your situation, we're here to share our experiences and to reassure you that everything you're thinking and feeling is normal.

- Filled with rage at how bloody unfair life feels right now? Normal.
- Ugly crying into your oat-milk flat white at the park? Normal.
- Haven't wept in weeks and wondering if you're even doing grief right? Also normal.
- Feeling a little isolated, and that few people understand what you're going through? Normal.
- Exhausted and overwhelmed? Yep, normal.
- Looking in the mirror and feeling like you've aged ten years? Pretty normal.
- Wondering why friends you thought would be there for you haven't shown up? You guessed it – normal!

Grief can make you feel like you're going crazy. It's messy and chaotic, and we all need a little bit of help to make sense of it. That's what we're here to do – to help you make sense of life after loss. We hope you find a little bit of comfort and understanding in the pages ahead, knowing that you're not alone.

Sal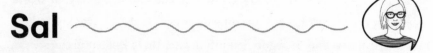

My introduction to grief came one morning in November 2019. I was brushing my teeth in my gym gear, ready to start my day, blissfully unaware that I was about to receive a phone call that would change my life. When the phone rang, it was my mum's partner, telling me that my kind, warm and caring mum, Rose, had died in the night from a sudden seizure (also known as SUDEP). 'I need you to steady yourself.

Your mum has passed away,' he said, as the words dripped down the line in what felt like slow motion. I ran into the bedroom to wake up my husband. 'My mum is dead. She's died. I don't know what to do,' I said in a state of sheer panic.

I'm from the UK but I live in Australia, and within 12 hours of learning of Mum's death, I found myself checking in at Sydney airport, trying to hide my tears as I prepared to board a 24-hour flight. I always knew the pay-off for living so far away was not being close if something terrible happened, such as a death. My worst nightmare had come true.

Grief is hard enough without having to fly solo over 10,000 kilometres to plan your mum's funeral! Life had flipped in an instant – I'd gone from sunny Australia to stepping off the plane into a UK winter, completely unprepared for what lay ahead. I was not only trying to wrap my head around the fact that my mum was dead, but I was also trying to grapple with jetlag, intense emotions and the endless admin that comes after someone dies. I wanted to fall apart, but there was no time for that. There was too much to get done and it was on me to do it.

In those initial months after Mum died, I was living on autopilot. My brain wouldn't let me fully comprehend the reality of what was happening – it would've been too much. I was under immense pressure to settle my mum's estate while I was in the UK and then also back in Australia, which caused a lot of stress. It wasn't until months later, when I finally had some breathing space, that the reality, and the sheer exhaustion, hit me (more on that later).

My mum was a real people person, curious by nature and incredibly compassionate. We had grown closer since I had moved to Australia and our relationship was moving into a new phase. Mum had become my confidante and we were starting to understand each other on a new level. It deeply hurts to think that, just as we were reaching a new place in our relationship, she was gone. To be honest, the whole experience feels shocking, even years on. I'm often struck with the thought, *How can a person who I have known my entire life, who knows me better than I even know myself at times, vanish from this earth without warning?*

Im

One drizzly Saturday morning in February of 2020, my mum Vanessa died by suicide. Argh. Those words on the page don't seem real, even years later. When I got the call, I was smack-bang in the middle of moving house with my nine-month-old baby in tow, removalists shuffling in and out. It was so surreal. I looked over to my baby and screamed, 'No. Not your grandma. This can't be happening.' I had been trying to call my mum all morning, but couldn't get through. I had an unshakable, heavy gut feeling that something wasn't right, but I could never have imagined her taking her own life.

That day will forever be a marker in time – a reference point for when my life was split in two: 'before Mum died' and 'after Mum died'. It was the day I began seeing life through an unfamiliar and catastrophic lens. Nothing has ever been the same since. There is now a huge Mum-sized hole in my life that will never be filled. Who will I text pictures of my aeroplane food to when I travel overseas? Who's going to nag me about going to the doctor when I have a cold? No-one cares about the mundane parts of your life as much as your mum. I lost my biggest cheerleader and my go-to support person for absolutely everything, and I miss her terribly. The sound of her singsong voice, her quirky op-shop presents that I pretended to love, and the way she used to get out her crappy little old paper diary from her zippy bag and hand write all her upcoming engagements. It's the silly little things we miss the most, isn't it?

Grieving my mum while simultaneously learning how to be a new mum myself has been a shitshow. I was just starting to get the hang of the 'tired new mum' gig when I became a 'suicide loss survivor'. Where do you even begin with that? Therapy, obviously! And lots of it. I'll be honest, the damage from my loss felt irreparable. Everything felt dark. For a long time, I wondered whether I was going to be able to find any light in my life again. (Spoiler alert: I did.)

HOW WE GOT HERE

As we both navigated our grief, living in the same city, we wondered if what we were experiencing was 'normal' or if we were going crazy (which we now know is a common thought many grievers have). We longed to connect with someone our age, who was also in the thick of grief, to ask them if they felt isolated, too. We were desperate to know if anyone else felt completely wiped out with exhaustion, couldn't think straight, or felt like a shell of their former self. We both yearned for someone who could relate.

One June afternoon, not even a year into our loss, we found ourselves in a pub garden in Sydney, searching for support. We had no idea that a brief encounter at a grief support group meet-up would change our lives forever. In the months that followed, we became fast friends. We instantly bonded over our shared experience of sudden loss and a mutual feeling of loneliness. We also have a lot in common (not just dead mums).

We laughed at the absurdity of the experiences we had been through since our mums died – the 'grief brain', the forgetfulness, and what not to do when scattering your loved one's ashes. We discussed how little Western society talks about loss and wondered how many other grievers were sitting at home feeling alone in their grief, too. (Turns out, a lot!)

Fuelled by our experiences, and a hope that we could help others feel less alone, we began the Good Mourning podcast. Our purpose is to create a space to talk about what grief is *really* like, telling it from the heart.

Good Mourning is your compassionate survival guide for all things to do with grief. It contains honesty, hope and a little bit of humour (we all need an extra dose of that when the chips are down). It's the support-group-in-a-book that we wish we were handed when our mums died, and we hope that it can be your compass as you navigate your loss. We're real, truthful, a little bit sweary, and on a mission to take the loneliness out of this hugely uncomfortable, yet universal, human experience. It's time to rip up the rule book on how we're supposed to 'do' grief, and have more open and honest conversations about loss.

WHAT YOU'LL FIND IN THIS BOOK

* **The experiences of others.** Sprinkled throughout these pages you'll find relatable stories and quotes from grievers of all ages, who have experienced all different types of loss.

* **Expert advice.** You'll find words of wisdom from our conversations with world-leading experts on grief and loss. We've also teamed up with psychologist Tamara Cavenett, who'll be sharing her professional opinion on some of the bigger topics we touch on. Tamara is immediate past President of the Australian Psychological Society (APS), the peak body for psychology in Australia, representing close to 30,000 psychologists nationwide.

* **Journalling prompts.** *Good Mourning* is more than a book, it's an interactive guide full of tools, writing prompts and exercises. Set aside a separate journal so that, when you come to a pen icon, you can jot down all your griefy thoughts and feelings.

* **The phrase, 'You are not alone.'** You'll hear this a lot . . . because we, along with thousands of others in this community, understand what you are going through and we are with you.

WHAT YOU WON'T FIND IN THIS BOOK

* **Toxic positivity. It's perfectly healthy to feel sad!**
* **Anyone telling you how you should (or shouldn't) feel.** Only *you* get to decide that.
* **A one-way ticket out of your pain** . . . because it literally does not exist (sorry!).
* **Silver linings. Sometimes crappy things happen,** for no good reason – death being one of them.
* **'At least . . . '.** Any sentence that starts with those two (annoying) words is banned here.

Whether your loss was recent, or it occurred many moons ago, we've learned that grief is a forever thing that changes shape over time. So, we've written this book in a way that you can pick it up and put it down, and take it at your own pace. Some of it may be useful right now, and other parts might make more sense later down the line. It's down to you and your loss – there's no 'one size fits all' approach when it comes to grief.

Although there's no 'bright side' to any of this, and reading this book won't magically make your pain disappear, we hope that it gives you insight and encouragement as you bravely learn to integrate your loss into everyday life.

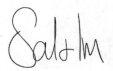

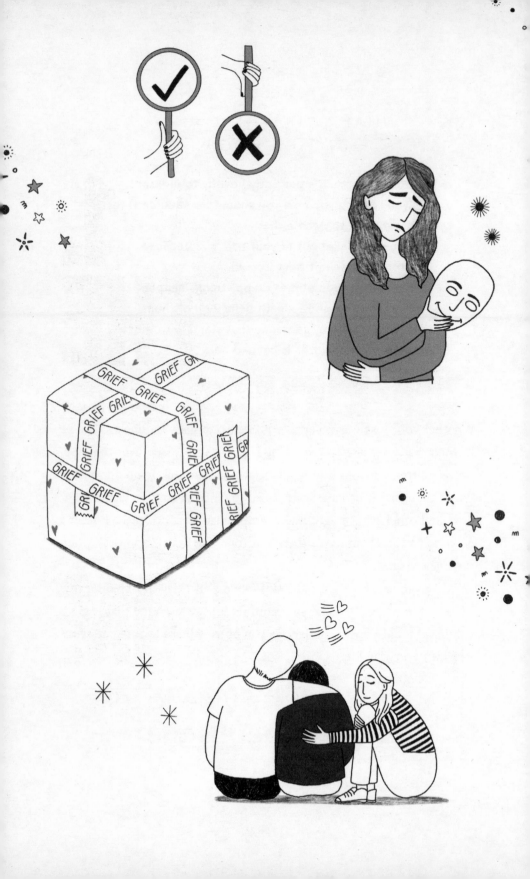

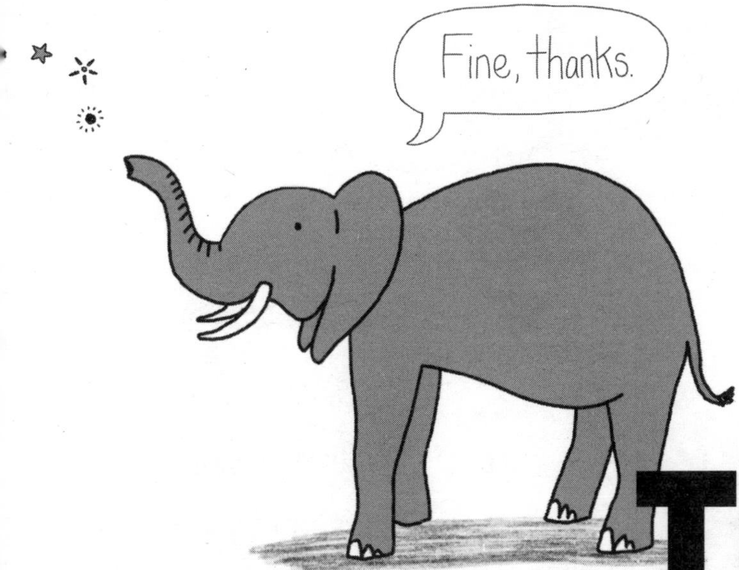

1. THE ELEPHANT IN THE ROOM

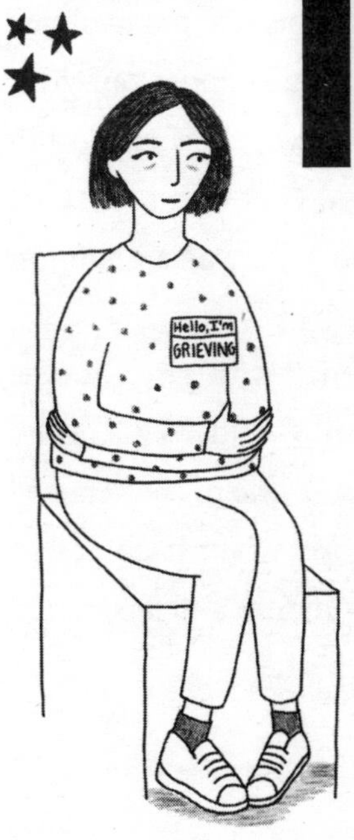

It's time to talk about grief

GRIEF IS AN EXPERIENCE FROM
WHICH NO-ONE IS EXEMPT,
YET WE'RE OFTEN COMPLETELY
UNPREPARED FOR HOW
CONFUSING, CONFRONTING
AND CRUSHING IT FEELS.

When we both became 'motherless' in our early thirties, we suddenly found ourselves in an unfamiliar and surreal situation that many of our peers couldn't fully understand. When we tried to talk about our grief with people who hadn't experienced loss themselves, it would often be met with an uncomfortable silence or awkward (but well-meaning) platitudes. 'Your mum wouldn't want you to be sad,' was a common one we heard.

People struggled to hear our honest experience with grief. It was isolating and lonely, despite having support from friends. This is the reason we decided to write this book, and probably one of the reasons you picked it up: people have no idea what to say when it comes to grief. So, even with the best intentions, they say random and misguided things in the hope that they will make you feel better.

The reality is that nothing anybody says is going to make you feel better right now. Someone in your life has died, you're in deep pain and life has upended – you're a million light-years from being okay. What you need is for the depth of your loss to be recognised and acknowledged. For someone to say to you, 'This is so shit and unfair. I know nothing I can say will take away your pain, but I want you to know that I am here. And I am not going anywhere.' If you don't have that kind of support in your life right now, rest assured that you are not the only one. There are way too many people grieving who are hiding behind a 'Fine, thanks', because it's easier than telling people the truth. It shouldn't be this way.

That giant, looming elephant in the room (aka your grief) that nobody wants to talk about needs to be acknowledged. We want to help make that happen. It's about time we shine a light on what grief is really like, one honest conversation at a time.

TALKING ABOUT GRIEF DOESN'T NEED TO BE AWKWARD

There are so many grief misconceptions and assumptions that fly around, and the expectations that people have, versus the reality, can be wildly off the mark. One of the biggest is that there are 'stages of grief' that you go through, which can be ticked off neatly and then life resumes. Not true! Others might assume that you should be 'over your loss' by a certain point and be getting back to 'normal' (whatever that is).

If your grief isn't recognised, or you feel like it must meet unrealistic expectations, it can make the whole process much harder to navigate. If anyone tries to tell you how you should be coping, or what you should be feeling, our advice is to please ignore them. And, if you're telling *yourself* any of this, please don't beat yourself up. You're coping with a hugely difficult life experience and, right now, you owe yourself bucketloads of understanding and the space to adjust, slow down and take things at your own pace.

Sal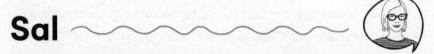

One thing that really surprised me about my grief was how, despite feeling deep pain and sadness, I was able to function pretty well. Of course, there were many moments when my emotions caught me off guard and I couldn't hold them in. Yet, in the early months, to the outside observer, I held myself together. Although I was heartbroken, the shock of the loss made it possible for me to cycle through the endless tasks and meetings, basically grieving via a to-do list.

While I powered through at work, in meetings and sometimes socially, on most weekends during the first year, I struggled to get off the sofa. It was almost like I was having a grief 'come down' from the week. But still, I judged myself and how I was processing my loss. Why was it that I could focus on practical things with a clear mind and get my work completed easily? Why wasn't I in floods of tears constantly, even though I felt sad? How come I could talk about my mum sometimes without getting upset? Was I normal?! The answer is yes. Being able to function most of the time doesn't mean you're grieving any less.

Im

On the contrary, my grief was absolutely debilitating and visceral. I was sitting on the other end of the spectrum to Sal, and I was also judging myself harshly. *Why can't I hold my shit together?* and *How come I'm unable to function like everyone around me?* were frequent thoughts I had. My grief has been an absolute clusterf*ck of overwhelming emotions. I would curl into a fetal position on the floor, howling for my mum. That feeling of her being ripped away from me forever was harrowing. Here I am, sobbing again as I write this. It doesn't leave you, does it?!

I was surprised at how physical my grief was, too. I was still breastfeeding my daughter when Mum died, and my body shut down. My milk supply completely dried up and I couldn't even feed my child anymore, which added another deep sense of loss. My skin felt like it was burning, and everything hurt. Some days, I honestly thought I was going to die from the pain.

When I was catapulted into grief, everything felt unfamiliar. Driving the car for the first time felt strange. Doing that first grocery shop felt wrong. The lights felt too bright, and I'd look around and see everyone going about their day as if everything was fine. It was the weirdest feeling. I was going through the motions of 'normal' life, but I felt anything but normal. I didn't feel safe in my body anymore and I desperately wanted to wake up and find out that it was all a bad dream.

Since Mum died, I've struggled with the constant feeling of there being something missing from my life. It's like a raw feeling of incompleteness, a homesickness. It's a pain that's hard to put into words, but if you know, you know.

What our community said about . . .

HOW GRIEF SURPRISED THEM

'I was surprised at how quickly you can go from having a great day to being absolutely crushed.'

'The shock of loss just "gets" you. You're okay one minute, and sobbing the next.'

'Even on days when I look happy and like I'm having a great time, I'm still in pain.'

'Grief is lonely, but my experience has made me much more compassionate.'

'I wasn't prepared for how awkward it makes even the most empathetic people.'

'I thought I was prepared because we knew the loss was coming, but I was not ready for how deep the pain is.'

'Ah, grief. It differs from person to person, even in your own family!'

Grief expectation

Grief reality

You stop grieving a few weeks after the funeral. → Grief lasts a lifetime (although it might ebb and flow over time).

There are set stages to grief. → There aren't stages that we go through. Grief is not linear!

Women feel grief more than men. → We all experience grief differently, no matter our gender.

You will go back to 'normal' eventually. → Grief can change you and your 'normal' might now look very different.

You're only grieving if you're crying. → Grief has many faces – sometimes it's visible to others, but a lot of the time it isn't. Not everyone is a crier!

Grief gets easier as time goes on. → Everyone is different, but sometimes grief can feel harder years into the loss, once the initial shock wears off.

You only need support during the first few weeks after a loss. → Sometimes, the months (even years) that follow are when you really need support, once reality sinks in.

Grief only comes after death. → There are many different things you can grieve, such as the loss of a job or relationship, estrangement, illness or injury (to name a few).

It is unhealthy to continue to talk about the person who died. → It's healthy and can be healing to talk about the person, for as long as you like.

THERE'S NO TIMELINE TO GRIEF

If you've found yourself on a grief-fuelled google search binge, it's likely you've already come across the famous Five Stages of Grief model, which was developed by psychiatrist Elisabeth Kübler-Ross in her 1969 book, *On Death and Dying*. The five stages she identified were denial, anger, bargaining, depression and acceptance, and these are often referred to as the benchmark steps for grieving. There can be an assumption that we can catapult through the five stages and be over our grief.

- ☑ DENIAL? TICK!
- ☑ ANGER? BEEN THERE, DONE THAT.
- ☑ BARGAINING? GOT THE T-SHIRT.
- ☑ DEPRESSION? NAILED IT.
- ☑ ACCEPTANCE? HERE I COME!

Oh, if only it were as simple as that. The truth? There's no set order to how you move through a loss, and it will encompass much more than these stages. It's not a straight line of stops, it's more like a big, black, messy squiggle. Some days you might feel deep anger and rage, and other days you might feel a glimmer of acceptance, only for that to be wiped away by a tsunami of denial. You can go through all five stages on the same day, in no order. And some days, you might feel nothing at all (also normal – more on that in Chapter 2).

Elisabeth Kübler-Ross referred to the five stages of grief as the 'five stages of death'. She came up with the stages when she was working with terminally ill patients, because these were common emotions she observed. The stages were never intended to be applied to the bereaved, and according to David Kessler, a world-leading expert on grief and the co-author of *On Grief and Grieving* (with Elisabeth), the five stages were not designed to be prescriptive. As he explained to us, they aren't linear – some people might experience all the emotions, some one or two and some none at all. There's no set order to the grieving process . . . and David's the expert on this, so he should know!

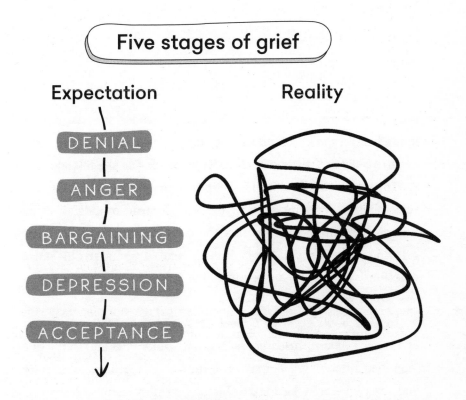

DOING GRIEF 'RIGHT'

So now we know that you don't have to get over your loss, you might be wondering if there's a 'correct' way to do this whole grief thing. However, there's no right or wrong way – our grief is as individual as we are. The way you respond to loss boils down to so many factors, including the role the person played in your life, past experiences, other life stressors, your mental health, cultural beliefs, and even your perception of death.

If you find you're deflecting unsolicited opinions or even comparing your grief to what others are experiencing, you might judge yourself negatively. Have you ever wondered if you're doing grief 'right'? Have you ever wondered if you're too sad, or if you aren't sad enough? Sal's coping mechanism is doing practical things (she's basically got a gold medal in it). So, she wondered why she was able to tick things off her to-do list and cope relatively well day to day. This ultimately led to questioning if something was wrong with her. Was she a robot unable to process emotions? Whereas Im, whose style is more 'curl into a ball on the floor and rock for days', gave herself a hard time for not being able to resume normal life as quickly as she felt she should.

There's no rule book on how to grieve properly (we ripped that up, remember?). You simply do it *your* way. Instead of judging yourself, it might be helpful to know that there are different coping styles for grieving. Like Im, you might be inclined to feel a strong range of emotions. Or maybe you're more like Sal and channel your grief by 'cracking on'.

In their book, *Grieving Beyond Gender: Understanding the ways men and women mourn*, researchers Kenneth Doka PhD and Terry Martin identified different grieving styles: 'intuitive' (aka feeling and expressing) and 'instrumental' (aka doing or taking a cognitive approach), which are the extreme ends of a spectrum. And it's very much a spectrum – they emphasised that you might find yourself leaning more towards one style, or you might be a blend of both (which is pretty common). Most people express grief in both doing and feeling ways, but, like us, you might find one style is a little stronger.

Kenneth Doka, explaining the styles, said that if you ask an intuitive griever about their experience of grief, they'll often talk about waves of emotion. Their expression of grief very much reflects what's going on internally, and they're likely to talk about finding support to explore their feelings, whether that's via therapy, a close friend, support group or creative expression, such as journalling. On the other end of the spectrum, an instrumental griever might show a completely different response to their grief, and be more likely to talk about it in a 'thinking' or 'doing' way. Their expression of grief could look like talking a lot about the person who died, or doing something in their honour, such as starting a charity fundraiser.

Intuitive grievers are more likely to:
- sit with and feel their emotions
- focus on processing their feelings and expressing them
- find strength and solace by sharing with others.

Instrumental grievers are more likely to:
- be more 'thinking' than 'feeling', taking a more cognitive approach
- focus on 'doing' by actively responding to their grief
- talk about their person (sometimes in a rational way).

Being aware of the spectrum can be helpful in understanding your way of coping with grief. Again, there is no one size that fits all!

For intuitive grievers, journalling, talking openly and finding peer support can be helpful ways of processing loss. Instrumental grievers might find healing by creating a legacy, planning a memorial, doing a problem-solving task, or talking about the person who died.

Kacie's experience with different grieving styles

'In April 2020, my life changed forever when my mum died of cancer. I'm an intensely emotional person who feels deeply, so it was no surprise to me that my grieving style is intuitive. I remember within the first few days crumpling into a ball in my kitchen, sobbing. I felt it in my whole body – the need to sob, to scream, to just talk about it. Knowing this about myself, I knew I needed to see a grief therapist. I have luckily found an amazing one who lets me cry as much as I need, explore and process my feelings, and helps guide me through the highs and lows that is the grief experience.

'My family has processed their grief very differently to me. My brother and my grandmother have more of an instrumental approach; their grief is inward and quiet. To me, as someone who needs to talk about my grief, their grief seems very absent. Not being able to easily share my grief with those who knew my mother best makes me feel lonely, and even angry at times. However, through the help of therapy and good friends, I have found ways to meet my grieving style outside of my family.'

What helped

'My advice for anyone who, like me, has family members who seem more absent or in denial, is to learn to let it go. It is not your responsibility to do anyone else's grief work; your load is heavy enough. Find friends or people in your life that you can trust and who will listen. And don't be ashamed to seek therapy – it's important to have a safe space to let it all out, especially if you're an instrumental griever. There is honour in putting your mental health first and finding someone who can guide you through grief.'

Think about how you've been coping with your loss and expressing your grief. Do you recognise yourself in the 'instrumental' or 'intuitive' grieving styles? Or, maybe you're a blend of both?

Your grief is

VALID

UNIQUE TO YOU AND
YOUR EXPERIENCE

AUTHENTIC TO THE
RELATIONSHIP THAT
YOU SHARED WITH
YOUR PERSON

Your grief is not

RIGHT OR WRONG

THE SAME AS
ANYONE ELSE'S

TO BE JUDGED
BY OTHERS

NO TEARS = NO GRIEF (JUST KIDDING!)

Have you experienced others assuming you are okay when really, you're far from it? Another grief misconception is that unless you're in floods of tears, then you're not grieving, or you're 'over it'. Not true – crying isn't a prerequisite for grief. It's common for people to internalise their pain to 'keep calm and carry on' (as we just explored with instrumental grievers). You may be functioning and look fine to others on the outside, but that is in no way a reflection of what is happening internally. There is a grief myth that looking okay means we are doing okay, but grief is often invisible, and you can't see a broken heart, but it doesn't mean that person isn't aching very deeply. You never truly know what sits behind a facade of 'coping' – grief is there, even if we might look fine on the outside.

People might ask, 'How are you?' and it can be easy to reply, 'Fine, thanks', because you're not sure if they're prepared for the real answer. You're probably feeling so flat, but outwardly it's easier to just smile and nod. And if people don't acknowledge your loss, or change the subject to avoid any awkwardness (more on this in Chapter 5), it can be hard to open up and be honest about what's going on inside. Sometimes, truth telling makes others very uncomfortable and you could be on the receiving end of remarks intended to try to 'fix' you, or lighten the mood. While it is likely meant as a kind gesture, the reality is that it's never helpful. You don't need cheering up right now – it's more than okay to feel incredibly sad. What you are going through is hard and your grief is not something that needs to be fixed. Please remember that.

Maybe we should take inspiration from Indigenous Australian culture, where there are signals to show others when you are grieving. Widows traditionally wore white plaster 'widow's caps' (also known as kopis) throughout the grieving period . . . no second-guessing there!

~~YOU'RE SO STRONG!~~

YOU DON'T HAVE TO PUT ON A BRAVE FACE. *It's okay to fall apart* **AND HAVE A BAD DAY. YOU'RE ONLY HUMAN.**

Jermaine's experience with being labelled as 'strong'

'My father died in 2014 and my mother died in 2015. I never expected to lose both of my parents so close together, and even though life had changed in a huge way, people often told me how strong I was for the way I was handling my grief.

'Because of this, I felt as though I was able to endure anything – I lost both parents and there I was, still standing tall. Being labelled as "strong" meant that I felt my grief was something I needed to have control over, or not show. What I really needed was a space where I could express my grief without fear or judgement.'

What helped

'I found peace when I allowed myself to grieve and feel my emotions without questioning my strength. I have learned that strength is not about how much pain you can endure, but instead recognising your feelings and not being ashamed to express them. Having a bad day doesn't make you weak.'

What non-grievers think grief looks like

What grief actually looks like

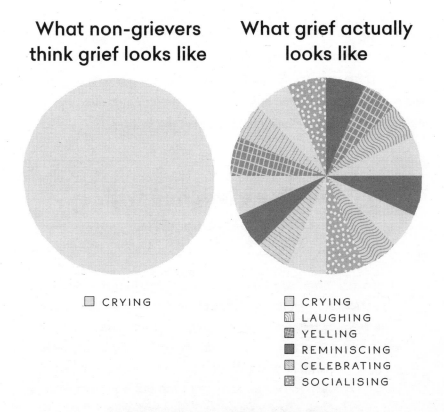

CRYING

CRYING
LAUGHING
YELLING
REMINISCING
CELEBRATING
SOCIALISING

ANTICIPATORY GRIEF

There's an assumption that grief only occurs after death, but that's simply not true. There's a type of grief that's super important to discuss, and that's anticipatory grief, which occurs *before* someone dies. It can be just as intense as the grief felt after death, no matter how prepared you are. Caring for someone who is terminally ill can be distressing, all-consuming and exhausting (both physically and emotionally). Seeing someone you love suffer is hard, and as they decline in health you might experience intense emotions, such as shame or anger. You may even feel a sense of relief, followed by guilt when they do eventually die. For some, knowing that death is imminent can bring on a state of anxiety or hyper-alertness, which is a huge energy drain.

Not only is it hard to watch someone you love in pain, you might also grieve for how it's impacting your life, too. When someone is dying, so many things can change and it can feel like you're grieving the loss of a future. It's normal to feel a mix of difficult emotions as you cope with an approaching death (more on this in Chapter 2).

Kelly's experience with anticipatory grief

'When my mum was diagnosed with Huntington's disease 18 years ago, I had no idea that I would feel grief before she died. Nobody told me what to expect and I was simply thrown into learning how to look out for my mum while simultaneously losing her. After 18 years of watching her slowly disappear, I am now aware that grief is so real even before death. From the moment you know it's coming, you're grieving. I liken it to feeling like you're always standing on the edge of a precipice. The pressure to stay strong and be there for the one losing their own life is constant.'

What helped

'I've learned that grief needs to physically move through the body. Whether that's through creative art, a walk outside or exercise, finding the thing that moved grief through my body was incredibly grounding for me. I've also learned to do more of the things that make me feel alive – because feeling alive includes all the big feelings, not just the happy ones.'

SECONDARY LOSSES CAN BE JUST AS PAINFUL

When you're grieving, you're not simply dealing with the tremendous grief from death loss, but also a multitude of smaller losses. These are called secondary losses, which can feel like curveballs and a painful addition to what is already a bloody difficult time. These 'non-death' losses might not always be obvious. However, their impact can be just as significant and can bring huge levels of stress to our lives because you're grieving not only the person, but also the huge hole they have left.

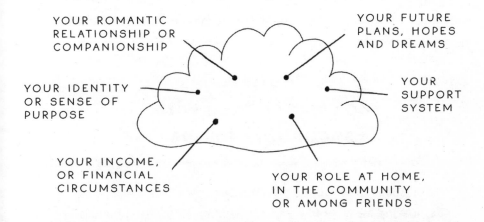

The unseen losses you're grieving

YOUR ROMANTIC RELATIONSHIP OR COMPANIONSHIP

YOUR FUTURE PLANS, HOPES AND DREAMS

YOUR IDENTITY OR SENSE OF PURPOSE

YOUR SUPPORT SYSTEM

YOUR INCOME, OR FINANCIAL CIRCUMSTANCES

YOUR ROLE AT HOME, IN THE COMMUNITY OR AMONG FRIENDS

Eleanor Haley and Litsa Williams, the duo behind the popular grief website What's Your Grief, describe secondary losses as being like a 'snowball effect', with multiple losses created from that one primary loss. The losses that come after a death gain traction and get bigger, compounding over time and impacting your sense of safety, confidence and wellbeing.

Because secondary losses can be situational and personal, they might not be as visible to others. People might not even realise that you are contending with other very big changes on top of loss, and that can be tough. Being 'non-death' losses also means that secondary losses are often seen as problems to be solved rather than things to be grieved. People might not see the different layers of grief you're wrapped up in right now and the added stress they cause. They probably won't write a sympathy card saying, 'I'm so sorry for the loss of your sense of identity' or 'My condolences on the death of your hopes and dreams, they will be sadly missed.' Although, maybe they *should*, as the loss of these things can feel just as painful as the death of our person.

It takes time to come to terms with all the changes. Allow yourself to have good and bad days. None of this is easy, but one thing that can help is practising accepting what *is*, without comparing it to what *was*. If you need some extra support, we recommend checking out the range of articles on secondary loss at whatsyourgrief.com.

Jo's experience with secondary losses

'My husband died suddenly from an asthma attack when I was 35, leaving me a widow and single mum to a four-year-old daughter. My entire world imploded – while my husband had physically gone, so much more went with him than I expected. Secondary losses are often not discussed, but they can be just as hard to cope with.

'When my husband died, I lost so much. I lost my best friend and confidant. I lost the father of my child, the person

I expected to parent alongside, and I lost my future. There will be no growing old together, no more children or marvelling together at the way our daughter has grown. In a way, I lost my past as well. He's no longer here to say, "Remember when . . . " and recall the incredible times we shared. I also lost my confidence – social situations became awkward; my identity had changed and the stability I once felt was no longer there. I lost my trust, because it's hard to trust the world when your life has been shattered and all you want to do is protect yourself from it ever happening again. There was not one aspect of my life that was not impacted by my husband's death. I was knocked so hard by the experience that I wasn't sure if I was ever going to get my life back again, but I did.'

What helped

'It's taken time, patience, support, and a great deal of inner faith when it comes to dealing with the loss of my husband and the secondary losses I've experienced. I see a psychologist regularly, am open about my experience and I ensure I do things for myself that bring me joy. The one positive about enduring such a huge loss is having a better understanding of what I want from my life and what is important to me, and empowering myself to have confidence in who I am now.'

Suzanne's experience with secondary losses

'In September 2020, I lost my 17-year-old son Samuel to suicide. Four months later, my mum died suddenly and two months after that, my dad died after suffering a stroke. That's three losses within seven months. Grief, funerals, probates, inquests and investigations became my life, all against the backdrop of a pandemic. I lived a surreal existence that I – let alone anyone close to me – couldn't comprehend.

'My three losses were the catalyst for myriad secondary losses. I suspected early in the grieving process that my relationship of six years was not going to survive. The support I received from my partner fell short of what I needed and deserved. He wanted the old me back, and I knew that person was gone forever. I withdrew to protect myself and couldn't envisage a future in this lonely and isolated place.

'Grief affected my confidence and identity, resulting in me withdrawing from friends and avoiding familiar places for fear of bumping into someone I knew. The risk of being confronted with their discomfort or sympathy heightened my anxiety. I reached a crossroads: I could either continue feeling isolated in a relationship, job and place that no longer served me, or I could make a change. I decided life was too short to put off making decisions. Within 18 months of Samuel's death, I left my career, ended my relationship, sold my home and moved 300 miles away to start afresh. Loss makes you appreciate how life can change in the blink of an eye. I lost a sense of fear as the worst in the world had already happened.'

What helped

'My advice would be to value yourself and your needs. If your loss feels like a catalyst for life changes, be brave and take baby steps. You deserve a future filled with meaning and hope that brings your loved one with you.'

NO NAMES MENTIONED

Talking about the person who died might sound strange to others, and there can be the assumption that even saying their name will upset us or remind us that they're dead – as if we could forget that! But in reality, it's quite the opposite, don't you agree? It's healthy to want to talk about your person. It's normal, and please don't let anyone tell you otherwise. We love it when people talk about our mums and ask questions about them – it means so much to us because it keeps their memory alive. There have been so many occasions when, on the tough days, sharing a story about our mums has given us a real lift, as it's a way to feel like they are part of our lives. Of course, it's different for us all – not everyone will feel strength from talking about their person, and that's okay. But if you do want to talk about them, know that it's healing to hear their name, to want to reminisce or share a story, because they are very much alive in your heart and mind. Just because their physical presence on earth is over, their impact on your life is not.

THE FIRST YEAR ISN'T ALWAYS THE HARDEST

Ah! The dreaded 'year of firsts'. During the first year of our losses, we were both under the impression that if we got through it – if we just made it through and survived – the worst was over. We were wrong. It takes time to learn to live without your person (and that's okay). It's different for everyone, but the one-year anniversary isn't the finish line for sadness. The first year can go by in a flash when you're consumed with shock, dealing with death admin (also known as 'dead-min'), or simply trying to readjust to a new life. It can be after the first year when the dust settles and the rhythm of life resumes that reality sinks in.

There's space between the time since you last heard your loved one's voice or felt their touch, making them feel further and further away. Years on, certain places, events or milestones can trigger grief. As time ticks by, your grief might not feel like constant pain, but it could still feel ever-present. It would be remiss of us to talk about the timeline of grief without acknowledging that sometimes people can feel as if they've come to a standstill and that there's no improvement in the way they feel as the months, or years, pass. If you're feeling stuck, or if you're finding that your grief is interfering with daily life for a prolonged period of time, and you are unable to function or take care of your basic needs, we recommend seeking professional help.

Psychologist Tamara's view on professional support

If you are struggling, it may be helpful to see a psychologist. There are a variety of skills and strategies that can be useful, such as mindfulness, acceptance and commitment therapy (ACT) and cognitive behaviour therapy (CBT).

It's important to note that grief differs from depression, which often requires professional treatment. Grief is associated with a specific event (the loss of a loved one) and the focus is on that loss. In depression, there is persistent and pervasive low mood and there isn't always an identifiable loss. It is important to note, however, that grief can morph into 'complicated grief', which can resemble depression in many ways.

Complicated grief is an all-consuming form of grief that happens when thoughts, feelings or behaviours that occur during grief interfere with the ability to accept the loss. With complicated grief, the response to a loss does not fade over time and can prevent you from getting back to daily functioning. Signs to watch out for include an inability to focus on anything but the loss, excessive avoidance of reminders, intense and prolonged feelings of sorrow or hopelessness, and an inability to resume daily life. A quick tip to try if you feel 'stuck' in your grief is to allocate 'grief' time – a pre-planned, specific time that's set aside for processing your loss. This can help you to function and concentrate during the other hours of the day.

Gina's experience after the first year of loss

'My dad died suddenly and unexpectedly in November 2019 when he was 67. The world went from being almost achingly normal to a dim version of itself. People would tell me that the first year is the hardest, but, actually, I started to feel everything in a much deeper way 13 months after Dad died. It was almost as if I was cushioned by shock and adrenaline during the first year.

'I remember thinking, I don't know what's harder, knowing that I have to carry on without him, or knowing I'll always be missing him. Because of this, I really don't like sitting still, because that is when the pain surges.'

What helped

'To help with the painful feelings, I focus on being creative. I write and paint and I also try to get outside every day for a walk or use my indoor bike for the days when I can't face going out. I can't say that creativity and exercise will always help, but they probably won't make you feel worse. Also, sometimes, you might do all the things you are "supposed" to do to help you, and still feel horrendous. And that's okay.'

What our community said about . . .

WHAT GRIEF FEELS LIKE
AS YEARS GO BY

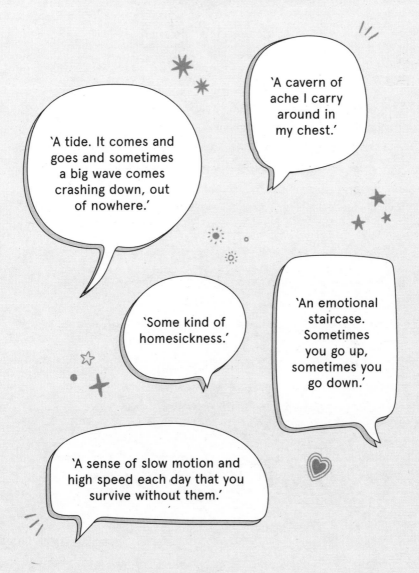

'A cavern of ache I carry around in my chest.'

'A tide. It comes and goes and sometimes a big wave comes crashing down, out of nowhere.'

'Some kind of homesickness.'

'An emotional staircase. Sometimes you go up, sometimes you go down.'

'A sense of slow motion and high speed each day that you survive without them.'

GRIEF NEVER GOES AWAY, BUT YOU WILL LEARN HOW TO *carry it.*

FLIPPING THE CONCEPT
OF CLOSURE ON ITS HEAD

As we move through the book, we want you to know there is no need to overcome your loss to find some form of healing. The idea of closure can be hurtful to some because, contrary to what non-grievers may think, we don't want to forget those who are gone. Some might assume that losing people means our relationship with them stops. Not true! Grief is learning to cope with major change, and it lasts a lifetime. It changes in intensity, but it is always there. It's how we learn to live with it that matters.

One of our favourite grief theories that backs this up is 'growing around grief', developed by Dr Lois Tonkin. You might have already heard of it because it's a popular theory, and rightly so. It helped us both reframe how we approach our grief. In her 1996 article 'Growing around grief: another way of looking at grief and recovery', Dr Tonkin suggested that grief isn't something you move on from, but something you learn to live with. She developed this theory after a woman, whose child had died, drew a diagram for her to explain how she expected grief to be. Instead of her grief shrinking, the woman's life grew around it and she learned to live with it as part of her. Her life felt bigger.

Over time, your grief might stay the same. But, instead of feeling as if you must shrink your grief to live your life, your life will begin to expand around your loss. It's a helpful theory because it relieves any pressure or expectation that your grief should have subsided by this point. Instead, accepting that grief is part of you can help you find peace and be able to live alongside it. We can move forwards with our lives, one baby step at a time.

Hope Edelman, author of the bestselling book *The AfterGrief: Finding your way along the long arc of loss*, believes that there's a big difference between what non-grievers think grief *should* look like and how it *really* behaves. The idea of closure is one example of this. As Hope explained to us, in Western society there seems to be a cultural imperative to have some sort of resolution or acceptance when it comes to loss. But, as you probably already know, grief isn't the same as a business deal. We don't just close it and move on.

Hope's view is that at certain points we may feel like we are leaning towards acceptance, but it's more like a train station that you arrive at, depart from and come back to at different points in your life. It's like a hub and a place that you move in and out of depending on your circumstances, but it's not a destination that is the end of the line. There's no finality to it. Our stories, she says, are always changing and growing as we learn new information and insights about the people who died, or we reach new planes of maturity. As she so wisely puts it in her book, the 'volume knob of distress' might get quieter over time and we might let in moments of joy or laughter, but it can 'amp up at key moments'.

We also spoke to David Kessler for his take on what 'acceptance' means, and he explained that people get confused with the concept, and think that acceptance means you're okay with death. But acceptance can simply mean that you acknowledge the reality. There isn't one big moment of acceptance – it's more like ongoing moments of acceptance you deal with. These can be big or small, like planning or attending the funeral, sorting out their belongings, selling the home you shared, eating at their favourite restaurant, or going to an event or experiencing a big milestone without them. All of these are continued moments of acceptance, no matter how big or small, and they may happen throughout our lives.

The 'grow around grief' theory

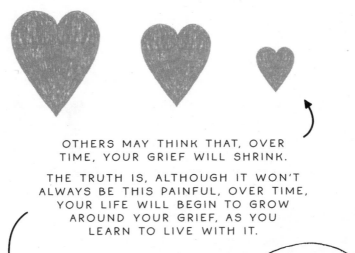

OTHERS MAY THINK THAT, OVER TIME, YOUR GRIEF WILL SHRINK.

THE TRUTH IS, ALTHOUGH IT WON'T ALWAYS BE THIS PAINFUL, OVER TIME, YOUR LIFE WILL BEGIN TO GROW AROUND YOUR GRIEF, AS YOU LEARN TO LIVE WITH IT.

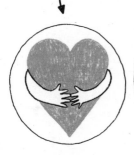 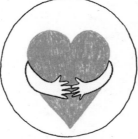 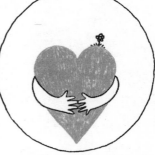

 GRIEF TIP

Let go of any belief that you must reach a final point with your loss in terms of acceptance, closure or moving on. You don't have to get over your loss – there is room for your grief to be part of you.

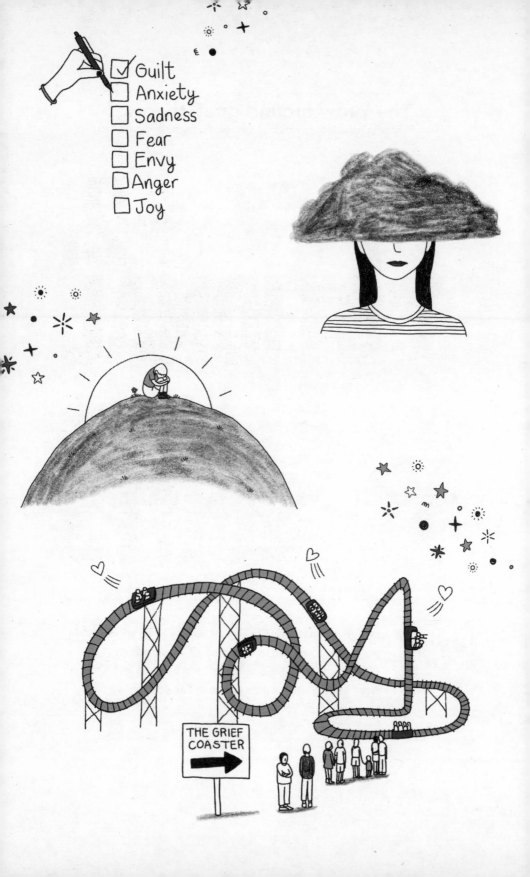

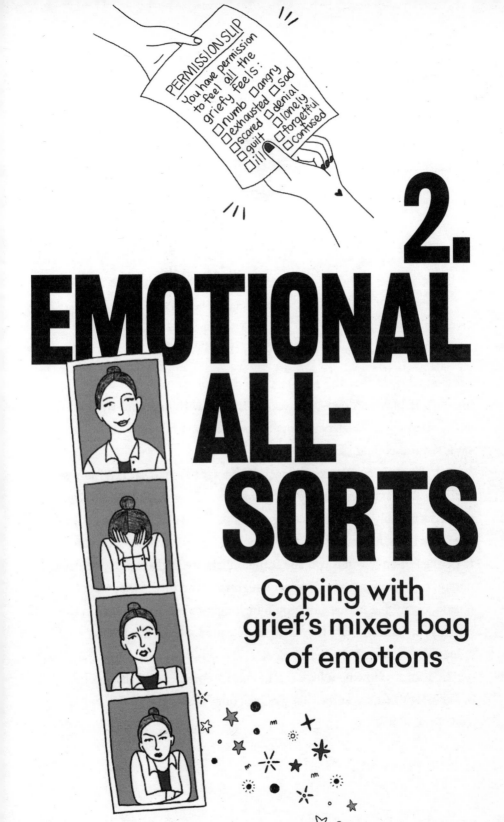

2.

EMOTIONAL ALL-SORTS

Coping with grief's mixed bag of emotions

DO YOU FEEL LIKE
YOU'RE AN EMOTIONAL
TICKING TIME BOMB?

Are you worried that the slightest pin drop of stress might trigger an uncontrollable meltdown? Are you so fuelled with rage that you could easily snap at the next person who looks sympathetically at you and says, 'You're coping so well!'?

People who haven't experienced loss might think that grief is just sadness. But, as you probably already know, it is so much more. Grief is uncontrollably sobbing because you miss someone so much and, in the same hour, hysterically laughing over a funny memory you shared. It's pangs of envy when you see someone else with their person – the person that you no longer have. It's regret for the things that were left unsaid, or missed phone calls you'll never get to return. It's fear in the pit of your stomach when you think of your future without them, or a deep yearning to hear their voice.

Emotions following a loss can be hard to predict and the intensity of them can make you feel like you're going crazy. You're not crazy – YOU'RE GRIEVING!

IF YOU FEEL OVERWHELMING
SADNESS, THAT'S OKAY.

IF YOU FEEL *full of anger,*
THAT'S OKAY.

IF YOU FEEL TOTALLY NUMB,
THAT'S ALSO OKAY.

IF YOU FEEL *regretful,*
THAT'S OKAY.

IF YOU FEEL A SENSE OF
RELIEF, THAT'S OKAY.

IF YOU FEEL NONE
OF THE ABOVE,
that's okay, too.

As deep as the feelings run, you don't need to hide them. The first step is to acknowledge that all the emotions you are experiencing, even the unpleasant ones, need to be felt. It can be tempting to block them out, but inviting them in is key.

Whether your loss is fresh or you're years down the line, you'll likely be feeling *all* the feels – sometimes all at once and sometimes not at all. One thing to remember is that although there's no finish line to grief, over time the emotional hurdles will begin to feel less frequent and your grief will become more manageable (as alien as that might sound right now).

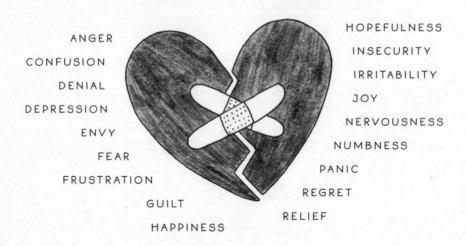

Grief can also feel like

ANGER
CONFUSION
DENIAL
DEPRESSION
ENVY
FEAR
FRUSTRATION
GUILT
HAPPINESS

HOPEFULNESS
INSECURITY
IRRITABILITY
JOY
NERVOUSNESS
NUMBNESS
PANIC
REGRET
RELIEF

What our community said about . . .

THE EMOTIONS THAT COME WITH GRIEF

'I am functional, and even though I have days where I feel anger and sadness, I am surprised at my ability to cope day to day.'

'I struggle with guilt on the days where I feel okay, as I think I should be feeling grief.'

'What emotions?! These days, I mostly feel numb.'

'I move between sadness and hope on a daily basis.'

'Before my sister's death, I had a handle on my emotions. Now, I feel angry almost all the time.'

'I feel an overwhelming dread that can make it hard to get out of bed.'

'Since my loss, I often feel overcome with envy.'

'Feeling irritated and frustrated has become a constant for me.'

'I have become hyper-sensitive and cry most days. Thanks, grief!'

It can be hard to regulate your emotions in the early days of grief. Know that this is normal. Next time an intense feeling hits, take note of it and name the emotion. It can help you to recognise what's going on for you.

ANGER: FIFTY SHADES OF RAGE

Anger is the unwanted guest at the party, the one with a bad reputation for swearing and seeing red. It makes others uncomfortable, so you might try to hide it or downplay its presence. But actually, letting anger in is okay. It's a healthy reaction to loss and it deserves a seat at the table.

When you're grieving, your temper could ignite for loads of reasons. You could be furious at the world for being so frighteningly unpredictable, at the unfairness of your situation, that no-one else around you seems to be going through the pain, or simply for the fact that your loved one has died and left you here to pick up the pieces. It's okay to be angry. Life has changed and none of this feels fair. But guess what? It isn't fair – you're allowed to be angry about that.

We spoke to Megan Devine, psychotherapist and author of the must-read book, *It's OK That You're Not OK*, and she told us that anger doesn't really get positive airtime in our culture. She's right – it's pushed aside. People recoil when faced with anger, because it's confronting and uncomfortable. But anger, as Megan explains, is a reaction to something that has happened to you that feels bloody unjust. So of course you are angry. Anger is *necessary*. She recommends seeing it as an energy to be expressed, rather than suppressed, and we agree.

The 'anger iceberg' metaphor is a helpful way to visualise what can influence anger. Developed by The Gottman Institute, led by Drs John and Julie Gottman, the anger iceberg describes anger as just the tip of the iceberg, shielding all sorts of unexpressed emotions lurking underneath the surface. Anger, in a way, is your body's defence to protect yourself from other underlying feelings. You might, unconsciously, express anger to deflect the raw emotions that lie beneath it. So, when you feel like you're at boiling point, it's a good idea to stop and ask yourself, *Is there anything else going on right now, underneath my pain?*

Here are just some of the other emotions that might be bubbling under the surface of anger. Can you identify with any of these?

- Insecurity
- Envy
- Sadness
- Hurt
- Fear
- Guilt
- Loneliness
- Shame
- Betrayal
- Worry
- Frustration
- Helplessness

Another good way to think of anger is as a vehicle to feeling better. Psychotherapist and grief expert Julia Samuel told us that anger is an expression of hurt, and finding ways to express it is how we heal. Blocking the pain can do you harm over time and limit your emotional bandwidth. If you allow yourself to feel the anger, including all the swearing and stomping that goes with it, it frees you up to begin to feel happiness and laughter again. Who couldn't do with a bit of that?

It probably feels like you're having to unlearn everything you know about painful emotions, but go with it. Give yourself permission to let the anger out. Here are some ideas on how to release the rage.

- **Hit up a boxing class.** And if that's not an option, punching or screaming into a pillow works a treat.

- **Go for a run.** Exercise helps to release pent-up emotions and gets endorphins pumping, which can boost your mood.
- **Breathe!** It sounds obvious, but deep breathing can calm your nervous system. There's a good reason people say 'take a deep breath' when someone is on edge.
- **Car scream.** Go for a drive and park your car somewhere secluded. Blast some music and then scream as loud as you need to, for as long as you like. It's incredibly cathartic.
- **Journal.** When you feel yourself reaching boiling point, grab your pen and vent.

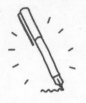

What emotions have been coming up for you lately? Have there been any feelings that have surprised you, such as anger? Take some time to write about what you've been experiencing. Remember, your feelings are neither good nor bad. They just are.

Paige's experience with grief and anger

'Following the loss of my nan and uncle within five months of each other, grief consumed my life and the waves of emotion varied day to day. Anger was a key emotion that I had rarely felt prior to my losses, and learning how to navigate it was tricky. It felt at times like a switch had been flicked and I found myself angry at the smallest inconvenience, such as something not going to plan, an email at work or an everyday discussion at home. In the early stages of grief, my family and I all went through the emotions at different times on different days – which is completely natural. Accepting this and trying to understand this together, while comforting each other, was just a small part of my grief journey, but a very important one.

'As the weeks passed by, I began to learn what I needed to do not only for myself, but for those closest to me. If I was having a really bad day, or could feel that anger switch waiting to be flicked, I would confide in my loved ones and even work colleagues, to let them know how I was feeling.'

What helped

'I made others aware that if I reacted in a different way to normal in a situation, it was not a reflection on them, it was just my grief. By doing this, family, friends and colleagues knew not to take anything too personally. This worked particularly well at home. My mum and I respected each other's griefy days and we knew when we needed to be left alone, when we needed a hug or even a good cry together.

'Something else I turned to was exercise. I was always the unfit one who paid for the gym and never went, but working out or going for a walk in the fresh air, releasing those endorphins, has played a huge part in my healing journey. So, whether you go for a run, do a 30-minute HIIT session or a long walk with your headphones on while listening to a podcast, take time for yourself to escape the "rage stage" as I call it. Appreciate what's around you and feel connected to your loved ones.'

GREEN WITH ENVY

Like anger, envy is an emotion that can feel incredibly uncomfortable – partly because it evokes a sense of being bitter or unpleasant, and sometimes even a sense of shame. However, envy is common in grief because, let's face it, life can feel unfair when suddenly there's a big piece of your puzzle missing. Everyday small moments can act as a trigger and a reminder of your loss, such as seeing someone with their partner, child, mum, dad, grandparent or best friend – it can be a reminder that you no longer have that, but other people still do. It hurts, like rubbing salt in a wound. There have certainly been times when we've been sitting in cafes or parks and feeling envious when we catch a glimpse of a mother and daughter having coffee, or grandmothers pushing a swing in the park. We've both felt that uncomfortable knot in the pit of our stomach, as we long to share even one last moment with our mums.

Envy is when you want something you don't have or, in this case, no longer have. In the context of grief, envy is an emotional response to loss. We are all human and envy is, in fact, part of the grieving process. It doesn't make you a bad person. It's not a 'wrong' emotion (because there is no such thing). In order to move through the feeling so that it doesn't morph into resentment, it is important that you acknowledge it, however uncomfortable that is. Something that helps us when we get a pang of envy is to stop and acknowledge it, because it's part of grief. Or we try to remind ourselves that although that person might seemingly have what we have lost, no-one truly knows what others are going through. It does the trick of helping to ease the feelings.

Psychologist Tamara's view on 'ugly' emotions

Grief feelings are often messy and complicated, and they can be ugly, too. People often call envy the 'lost stage of grief'. It is perfectly normal to experience anger, resentment, bitterness or envy as part of grief, and it takes a great deal of courage to admit to those parts of ourselves about which we're not proud.

Try not to judge these darker emotions; all feelings are okay. You cannot control your thoughts or the way you feel, only what you do with those feelings. We are human, none of us are perfect and feelings serve a purpose. It is reasonable to feel envious that someone else gets to live or to have experiences that you may not get to enjoy. It can be helpful to share these feelings with a trusted person who has also been through a loss.

Recognise and acknowledge your thoughts, and accept your feelings. Allow yourself to experience the emotions without judging or suppressing them. For example, tell yourself that it's perfectly expected to feel envious and angry that a friend will get to have an experience that you miss having.

It's important to remember that we often feel conflicting emotions. You can feel envy while still not directly wanting the other person to also suffer the loss that you are feeling. It can be helpful to reframe your thoughts. The 'dark' emotions you are feeling are actually a sign of how significant that loss is for you, and the depth of that pain. It can be helpful to also separate feelings from behaviour – you can still behave towards the person in line with your values, all the while experiencing feelings such as envy or bitterness.

Fiona's experience with envy

'In 2019, my husband drowned in a work accident. He was 29 and I was 26 at the time. He went to work one morning and never returned. The first few weeks were a blur, getting affairs in order and arranging the funeral. As the weeks progressed and I returned to work, everyone else's lives around me went back to normal, even though my world hadn't. It was around this time that I felt very envious of other people's lives and relationships – friends and work colleagues; I even found my parents' marriage to be almost triggering. Everyone else still had their person to do life with, while mine was ripped away from me before we even had a chance to really start our lives together.

'I would constantly see couples or families walking down the street and be envious that they had their person to hold hands with, to talk about their day and just be in each other's company. A moment that really sticks out in my memory is when I was sitting with my friends discussing my late husband and my grief, and they said that they were home last night talking to their own husbands about my grief and losing their friend. I felt an overwhelming sensation of envy and anger that they had someone to go through their grief with, and that I was sitting alone to deal with mine. I couldn't cope with any couples fighting or whinging around me, either. I often thought about what I would give to even have one last fight with my husband, or to just hear his voice again.'

What helped

'I began writing a letter to my husband each night, as a way to pour out my heart and soul to someone. I would tell him about my day, how I felt, the things I mourned that we couldn't experience in our future, or what was happening with his family. I've never read back what I wrote in those letters, and I've never let anybody else read them either, but writing them allowed me to feel a connection with him. For anyone else struggling with feelings of envy, I recommend writing to your person. It helped me keep a connection in my relationship and see the beauty again in other relationships, rather than letting my feelings overwhelm me.'

What our community said about . . .

DEALING WITH ENVY

'Sometimes, to put it into perspective, I think about how other people could easily be envious of me. I'm envious of people who have their parents alive after 21 years because I don't, but somewhere out there, someone may be envious of me that I got to have my parents around as a child and teen.'

'Working out is a great outlet, I have found. Punch that envy away!'

'I give myself the time and space to feel the emotion. I don't push it aside.'

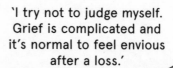

'I try not to judge myself. Grief is complicated and it's normal to feel envious after a loss.'

'I shamed myself for feeling envious, until I realised it is something that so many other people feel, too. Now, I don't feel bad when the emotion arises.'

'I acknowledge my feelings but try not to let them eat me up.'

'I always tell myself, *You're envious of someone, but remember they may only appear to have who or what you want. You never know the full story of their life.*'

'A social media break helps with feelings of envy. I know I've been scrolling for too long when I start feeling envious of other people's relationships.'

'If I get triggered, I go and treat myself to something that I know will make me feel a little bit better.'

GRIEF AND GUILT (AKA 'THE GRUILTS')

Have you spent far too many hours ruminating on all of the things you should've, would've and could've done differently? Are you fixated on replaying every time you upset your loved one, weren't a perfect person and said or did things that you didn't mean in the heat of a moment? If you're internally screaming, *Yesss! Guilty!*, you, friend, are not alone.

Guilt feels like such an inescapable companion to grief that we coined a term for it: 'the gruilts'. It's brutal and all-consuming at times, and can feel like a heavy weight. It's your mind's answer to where to lay blame – thinking that the outcome could be different if only you had changed your actions.

It's important to point out that guilt is not just felt after a death. People experiencing anticipatory grief when caring for someone at the end of life are often emotionally exhausted by watching someone they love decline in health, or die without dignity. There can be guilt for harbouring these feelings or for wanting to stop watching their loved one suffer. You may even feel a sense of relief when your loved one does eventually die, followed by feelings of guilt for feeling that way. This is a normal and natural reaction, and comes from a place of love.

If you are familiar with the gruilts, could you do us a favour? Please bookmark this page, so that on those guilt-riddled-grief days when you get sucked into the spiral of self-blame, you can repeat these four words: IT'S NOT MY FAULT.

Go on, say them out loud and say them over and over again, as many times as you need to until they sink into your psyche. Because it really isn't your fault. We know this won't take the pain of your guilt away entirely, and what you need right now is for your complicated thoughts and feelings to be validated. But we want to gently remind you that feelings of self-blame after loss are normal.

Im

My mum didn't leave a note. I had no answer as to 'why' she died. So, I conducted my own 'psychological autopsy' to try to determine what happened. In the process, my mind would grasp onto thoughts that perhaps it was all my fault. *Why couldn't I have saved her? Why wasn't I enough to keep her here? What if I'd called her 30 minutes earlier? If only I saw the signs!* It was debilitating. I would ruminate on every single word exchange in the months leading up to the day. I was so fixated on all the details and hopeful that if I could come up with a narrative that made sense, then perhaps it would either bring her back or, at the very least, take away this added layer of pain. Unfortunately, every path led to the same dead-end of disappointment. No answer served me that sense of relief I was so desperately searching for. I was riddled with guilt and regret.

We spoke to actor and breast cancer awareness advocate Samuel Johnson, who has had three people close to him die by suicide. I asked him how he gets up and faces each day after experiencing such tragedy, and he told us that the most important thing with suicide is not to ask, 'Why?', because the answer is always the same: at that point, life was too painful. I find it really helpful to reflect on Samuel's perspective when those feelings of self-blame start to resurface.

When I can feel my guilt spiralling, I practise shifting my focus to an earlier, more positive memory of my mum. She is so much more than the way she died. We were extremely close, and her death was just one moment out of 32 years of a loving connection. We can often get stuck focusing on what we didn't do, or what we felt we should have done around the time of someone's death, that we lose sight of all the loving and wonderful things that we did for them throughout the entire relationship.

Sal

I relocated to Australia in 2014. Since Mum's death, I've felt massively guilty for not being geographically closer to her in the years before she died. On top of this, the last time I saw her was nine months before she passed, when she'd been in Australia visiting me. Towards the end of her trip, I was ready for some space. I remember practically bundling her into a taxi to the airport, not knowing it would be the last time I saw her alive. This memory would replay and I'd ruminate on it, overcome with regret and feeling like a terrible daughter.

I wished I could turn back the clock and say a proper goodbye, but, of course, that wasn't possible. And so I had to find a way to process these guilty feelings and thoughts. I remind myself that guilt is a normal response to death and that I wasn't wrong for needing a breather. I didn't know it would be the last time I saw my mum alive, and I had to cut myself some slack. Journalling has helped me process these thoughts. Instead of focusing on the last time I saw her, I write about, and reflect on, all the times we spent together.

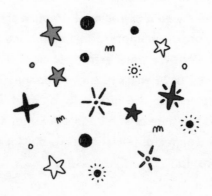

Priyanka's experience with survivor guilt

'After my baby girl Lily died at ten months old, I was plagued with survivor guilt. No parent should ever have to bury their child. I suffered from guilt that I couldn't save her, guilt that her disease was terminal, guilt that I had to give my baby such strong drugs and guilt that I am still here and she's not. The hardest thing about regrets when someone has died is that you don't get a second chance. You can't wake up and try again. While hindsight is a torturous thing, I work through my feelings by reassuring myself that no matter how much I want to, no amount of guilt will change the past.'

What helped

'When guilt comes to call and it feels dark, I have learned to trust in myself that I made the best decisions based on all the information I had at that time.'

What our community said about . . .

GUILT AND REGRET

'I didn't see my dad in person for 18 months before he died, as I was busy living my new life overseas. It was only a two-hour flight home. I have so much guilt for not going back more. I also missed his last call, two days before he died. I would do anything to be able to answer it now.'

'When my sister died, I constantly went over the things that I could have done differently to try to prevent it from happening. *What if I had done this, what if I had done that?* It's exhausting.'

'My aunt passed away and I wish I'd spent more time connecting with her while she was alive, as only now, through others' stories, am I realising how alike we are.'

'I struggle with the guilt of forgetting my brother. The guilt of moving on with life. The guilt of making new memories. The guilt of experiencing the things he would've loved. The guilt of still needing him for my own self-serving reasons. It feels like it never ends.'

'I was my mum's primary caregiver and responsible for making all her medical decisions. I am constantly worried about whether I made the right choices at the end of her life. It's so hard to get out of the guilt cycle.'

'My dad passed away suddenly. His birthday was two days before he died, and our phone call was cut short. I said I would ring him back but never did. I feel so guilty.'

Erica's experience with guilt

'My mother suffered from diabetes and in early 2011 her health started to decline. The relationship that my siblings and I had with our mother was complicated – over the years we did what we could to help take care of her, but as time went by, the relationship became more strained and distant. I eventually removed myself for the sake of my mental health and, while I didn't have any regrets at the time, since her passing I have felt tremendous guilt.

'I have frequent thoughts of *I should have done more, I could have been more present,* and *I should have put up with the constant fighting – she was going through a lot.* My mother wasn't pleasant to be around, so I became distant. After her passing, I would often hear "she was sick and lonely", "she needed you girls", and my guilt continued to grow. My mother lost her own mother at a young age and she did not allow herself to grieve. I believe that is a large contributing factor to the strained relationships she had within our family. As I continue to navigate my own grief, I am beginning to realise how difficult it probably was for her and it makes me wish I could go back and do things differently.'

What helped

'There are a couple of practices that have helped me with the grieving process, and one is that I have built a strong community of people I can talk to about my thoughts and feelings around the loss of my mother.'

Managing guilt and regret

Here are some ways you can manage feelings of guilt on tough days.

- First up: forgive yourself!
- Remind yourself as many times as you need to that guilt is a normal response to loss.
- Don't be afraid to share your thoughts and feelings (however irrational they may seem) with a trusted friend, family member or therapist.
- Remind yourself that letting go of your guilt does not mean letting go of your loved one.
- Think of the positive things that you did together. Write them down so you can read them back on days when you feel guilty.
- Write a letter to the person who died, explaining the thoughts and feelings you're experiencing. Getting it all out on paper can be a helpful way of releasing guilt.

WHEN THE RELATIONSHIP WAS COMPLICATED OR ESTRANGED

Relationships can be complex. Even the very best ones can be challenging at times, but when someone dies and your relationship wasn't in a good place, or it was estranged or ambiguous, it can bring up unanswered questions, mixed thoughts and feelings, or even a sense of relief.

Sometimes, there's no chance to resolve complications before someone dies, or the desire to make amends might not have been there. In truth, not every loss is mourned. We often refer to the person who died as a 'loved one', but perhaps you didn't love them. Perhaps you don't miss them. That's okay. Even when the relationship was estranged or complicated, you can still feel deep grief and mourn for the loss of the relationship that you never got the chance to have.

You may experience feeling:
- shame around being relieved about their death
- lonely and unable to express your grief with others because you didn't have a 'good' relationship
- guilt and regret that you didn't mend the relationship or make contact before they died
- surprise from unresolved feelings that surface, that you thought would disappear when they died.

Whatever you are feeling – however complicated – your emotions are valid. If you are left with unresolved issues, or feelings that have been left unsaid, here are some ways you can work through them.
- Name the emotions as they arise. Write them down.
- Write a letter to the person. Tell your truth and let it all out.
- Find a therapist you can work with to help resolve your complicated relationship.
- Find forgiveness for yourself or for the person who died. It isn't about excusing any wrongdoings of the past, it's about freeing yourself from any strong emotions you may be holding onto that are impacting your ability to move forwards with your life.

WHAT TO DO WHEN A GRIEF BOMB STRIKES

You may have heard of the well-known analogy of the 'waves of grief', when strong feelings wash over you. We like to call them 'grief bombs' – life can feel like a minefield of emotional triggers and reminders of your loss, which can land out of nowhere when you least expect it.

Picture this: you're walking down aisle five in the supermarket and you get a whiff of your person's aftershave or perfume. Maybe you spot their favourite biscuits. It could be something small or random that takes you to a memory of them, but – *BOOM* – just like that, you're back at day one with gut-wrenching, head-spinning and inconsolable grief. Your world comes crashing down all over again. 'How could they be gone?' you whisper to yourself as you abandon your trolley and run for the nearest exit, too embarrassed to be seen wailing in public. We've both been there, *many* times.

Sal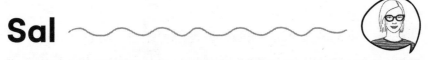

One of my most vivid memories of a grief bomb hitting was when I was in an Uber with a work colleague, heading to dinner after a big event. The mood was celebratory as it had been a great day. Then, the song 'High' by Lighthouse Family came on over the car speaker. It was Mum's main funeral song and the one that is most difficult to hear. I panicked – one minute I was smiling and laughing, the next I was completely uncomposed and sobbing. It was as if I was right back at the crematorium, saying goodbye to her.

Im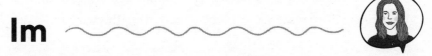

A big trigger of grief bombs for me is grandmas. Sweet, harmless, little old ladies with their grandkids – hardly what you'd think would cause a cascade of emotion! One day, when I dropped my daughter off at day care, a lady was at the door saying goodbye to her granddaughter who was around the same age. She held the door open and doted over my daughter. Emotions were exploding inside of me. I tried to hold it together until I could run back to the car and let out uncontrollable, body-shaking, snot-dripping sobs.

Adjusting to your 'new normal' without your person is incredibly difficult, bombs and all. It's no wonder that even years after your loss, the thought of them being gone forever can still take your breath away. Although grief bombs will hit with less frequency over time, they won't disappear entirely. But, if you allow yourself to feel them when they hit, as exhausting as they are, you might feel a smidgen lighter afterwards.

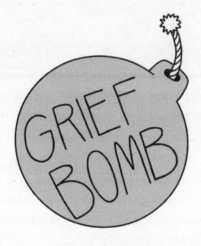

WHEN EVERYTHING SEEMS TO BE
OKAY, THEN OUT OF NOWHERE
THE GRIEF HITS, LIKE A BOMB
EXPLODING IN YOUR HEART

GRIEF TIP

If you're in a situation where a grief bomb strikes and you're around others, be open and honest about what's happening. Don't be afraid to be vulnerable and let others support you.

What our community said about . . .

WHEN GRIEF BOMBS
HAVE HIT THEM

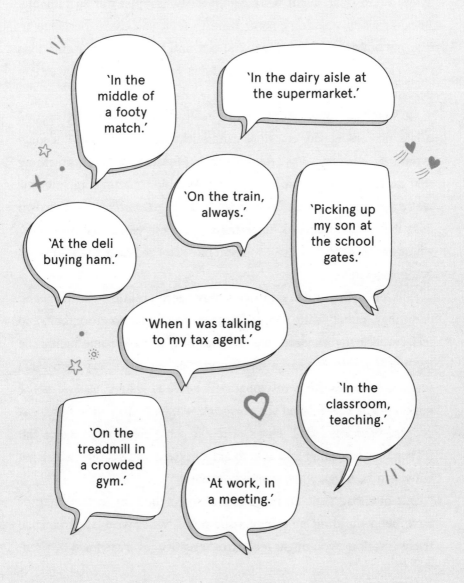

FEELING IS HEALING

Let's take a moment to talk about avoidance. When life gets busy, you might think you don't have time to grieve properly. 'NO TIME TO CRY' might be your slogan as you keep on going and push your feelings aside. While that might work temporarily, it's just not sustainable. Because when you don't make time to feel, you can experience an internal build-up of emotions. You can only shrug off your emotions for so long before they spill over and demand to be felt, and your cup becomes full, brimming with pain.

It sounds so obvious, but crying really does play an instrumental role in processing your emotions in a healthy and healing way. But some avoid it at all costs. Why? Because crying forces you to be something that can feel innately uncomfortable: vulnerable (instrumental grievers, we're looking at you!). In her book *Daring Greatly*, Brené Brown describes vulnerability as 'uncertainty, risk and emotional exposure', which are three things that can seem like giant red flags to avoid when you're grieving.

Sitting with painful emotions may seem counterintuitive (and daunting), but allowing yourself to step out of your comfort zone, and feel emotionally exposed, has been proven to have some incredible healing benefits. Research has found that when you cry emotional tears, it activates the parasympathetic nervous system, as well as the region of the brain called the amygdala, which helps you to relax *and* process your emotions. Think of it like a big clear-out, leaving you feeling lighter, calmer and able to get a better night's sleep (which we know can be tough when you're grieving).

All of those pent-up feelings we've touched on in this chapter have been building up inside your body. When you don't release these emotions, you might feel extra sensitive, overwhelmed or tired.

These are all good indicators that it's time to let yourself be vulnerable. Allow us to introduce you to the 'grief sesh'.

The grief sesh

The grief sesh is *the* secret weapon for unblocking the heavy emotions on really hard days. It is when you actively force yourself to grieve by provoking an emotional release. Here's how it works.

A step-by-step guide to having a grief sesh

Firstly, you will need a toolkit. Everyone is different, but for some inspiration, here's what's in ours:

* music that reminds you of your person
* photos – *allllllll* the photos!
* handwritten cards or letters from them
* their journals
* items of jewellery of theirs and clothing that holds their scent
* a pillow to scream 'fuuuuuuuck' into
* tissues and a glass of water.

NOTE: Before we dive in, we want to flag that this exercise can bring up a lot of painful emotions and if you are someone who tends to suppress your feelings, accessing these emotions can feel overwhelming. If it feels too much for you, you can come back to this exercise when you are more likely to be emotionally ready. There is no rush.

STEP 1 Find a cosy, private space where you won't be interrupted (this is key – we've been interrupted mid-sesh and it can be awkward!).

STEP 2 Music is an integral part of a good grief sesh, so play some music that reminds you of your person. The funeral songs work a treat, or you could listen to their favourite albums. You could also create your own 'grief sesh playlist' on Spotify that evokes memories of them.

STEP 3 Take a deep breath. Listen to the music while you look at photos or read cards, letters or journals. Hold the special items, smell their clothing and accept whatever emotions arise, without judgement. Use the pillow if you want to have a good scream – try not to hold back or suppress whatever comes up for you. Remember, by doing this, you are helping to process the pain that has been living in you rent-free. Take as long as you need.

STEP 4 When you feel like you've had a good cry, or that you've managed to express some of the feelings inside, stop. And be sure to go easy on yourself afterwards. You can feel exhausted after a grief sesh so try to keep your schedule clear for a few hours to rest and recoup.

Next time you feel like you're bottling up your grief, have a sesh. Whatever you've been holding tightly in your vault for fear of losing control, let it out. You'll be surprised at how much of a relief it can be to allow yourself to feel.

While it's good to get the feelings out, it's important to acknowledge that sometimes you *don't* feel all these emotions. You just feel numb. We've experienced this, too, and it's perfectly okay. The initial months or even years can be clouded by shock. When we spoke with the incredible author and grief advocate, Jo Betz, she described the first year of loss after her husband died of an asthma attack as being like some sort of survival game show. She was powered by adrenaline and shock. The big emotional hit for her came at the one-year mark of her husband's death. She thought that if she could do everything 'right' in that first year, she might be able to 'beat' the grief. She turned up to every social event and threw herself into work, only to realise that there was no real reward waiting for her when she got to the finish line. It was only then that the big emotions began to surface.

So, if you aren't feeling all the feels, no matter how long it's been, know that this can be a common experience. There's nothing wrong with you, and the feelings might come in time.

TAKING A BREAK FROM GRIEFY FEELINGS

On the topic of avoidance and processing feelings, you need to be able to have a bit of a break from the constant hit of emotions, and there's a theory that backs this up. The Dual Process Model was presented by Margaret Stroebe and Henk Schut in a paper called 'The Dual Process Model of Coping with Bereavement'. What makes this model so interesting is that it challenges the myth that grieving requires you to only focus on grief. Instead, it suggests that you might actually be able to cope better by having time where you don't think about all your griefy feelings. Instead of grief being something that is faced head-on all the time, the model suggests that there are two main 'stressor' modes that grievers can operate between: loss-oriented stressors and restoration-oriented stressors.

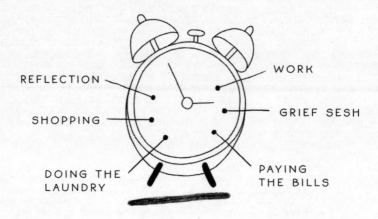

REFLECTION

WORK

SHOPPING

GRIEF SESH

DOING THE
LAUNDRY

PAYING
THE BILLS

Loss-oriented stressors are things like working through your grief, or scheduling in a grief sesh. On the flipside, restoration-oriented stressors are things that you might have to do in everyday life, like paying the bills, cleaning the house, being present at work or shopping for food. A big part of the concept is the idea of oscillating between the two stressors – Stroebe and Schut say that people switch back and forth between them as they grieve. For example, you might be crying in the toilet one minute and then go back to dinner with friends the next. Without a little restoration-oriented behaviour, and a bit of a break from the intense emotions, it would be hard to get on with daily life. Moving between the two helps you focus on the day to day, while also tackling emotional stressors as they pop up. While it is important to take the time to feel your emotions, know that it's also normal to give yourself a break and focus on other things.

GRIEF AND JOY: A PECULIAR DUO

We've spent a lot of time looking at the hard emotions that accompany grief, but it doesn't always have to be doom and gloom. Positive emotions can (and will) live alongside your pain. Grief cracks you right open and, in the darkness, there have to be some moments to let a little light in. The problem is, when someone dies, joy can feel like a swear word. It doesn't matter where you are or what you're doing, the pain inside hurts so deeply that it can feel inappropriate to experience happiness or excitement. However, it would be overwhelming to feel consumed by grief at every moment. Instead, maybe you'll find little pockets of happiness, even on days when you least expect it. Although the loss will remain, there can be room for joy.

Joy might simply mean savouring the little pleasures in a day. Smelling a flower. Sitting in the sunshine. A moment of laughter with a friend. Getting lost in a good book. Eating a slab of chocolate and feeling satisfied. Going for a run. You get the drift? Making time and space to let joy in can be as easy as setting aside a few minutes for yourself each day that allow you to feel a little pleasure.

What helps Sal: Spending time in nature, with either a walk along the beach or a swim in the ocean. Immersing yourself in the outdoors and getting fresh air can boost your mood.

What helps Im: Bingeing *Schitt's Creek* on Netflix – laughter is medicine.

It's okay to feel moments of joy – it doesn't make you a bad person, or mean you aren't grieving. Grief is a mixed bag of emotions. Remember, however you feel is right for you. What someone else experiences might not be the same as what you experience. Let go of any judgement of yourself.

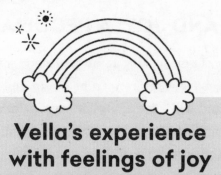

Vella's experience with feelings of joy

'I unexpectedly lost my mother on 16 October 2020. In the midst of the global pandemic, I was absolutely devastated. I had to travel back to my home state and that also took a mental toll. When I arrived back home, my dad and siblings were all waiting for me, and we embraced one another and cried. Although I was drained emotionally and physically, the following day we met our extended family at my uncle's house. As we reminisced and laughed about Mum, it felt great to laugh and be with my family, but then I immediately felt guilty about feeling anything other than utter sadness.'

What helped

'I very quickly learned that it is okay to laugh and feel happiness and light-heartedness in the middle of grieving. There was no need for me to feel guilty. My mum would have been proud of us for not letting her death completely consume us and for finding a way to continue to live and laugh. I try to remind myself of that always, and I feel her with me when I'm remembering her and smiling.'

What makes you feel a little lighter on the rubbish days? Is there something that you used to do that brought you joy before losing your person? It might be really simple – something like connecting with a friend or making time for exercise. Write down three things you could do to bring a glimmer of joy on extra-griefy days.

FINDING HOPE WHEN YOU'RE FEELING HOPELESS

It can be hard to imagine anything good coming from the death of someone you love. When you're grieving, it's not easy to see brighter days ahead. We understand.

Although death is shit and there's no amount of glitter that we can sprinkle over the situation to make it better, sometimes holding onto a little hope can help you reframe how you feel about living with grief, and you might even discover that you have more resilience than you think. Psychotherapist Julia Samuel shared some sage advice about hope with us. She explained that hope isn't just an emotion, it's also a plan. A plan on how to make your way forwards after loss by setting realistic goals, and believing that you can make them happen. She says that even if you have the tiniest flicker of hope, it can make all the difference.

Another perspective on hope that has helped us both comes from Dr Edith Eger, a Holocaust survivor, psychologist and author. She shared with us how when she was sent to Auschwitz at age 16, she was able to find it within herself to choose hope, even in the most unimaginable circumstances. Her solace came from discovering an internal strength, realising that the words inside her head made a tremendous difference in her ability to maintain hope. She explained that if you change your thinking, you can change your feelings, and that we all have the capacity to choose hope. We don't get to choose what happens to us, but we do get to choose how we respond to our experience, and shifting our focus to thinking about hope, rather than hopelessness, is a great place to start. Her stance on hope during difficult times is a realistic one, too – she says you don't have to overcome your loss; you just have to come to terms with it.

On the topic of changing your thinking, a useful tool that can help you cultivate a more hopeful mindset is cognitive reframing. It's a popular technique that's used in cognitive behavioural therapy (CBT) to reframe negative thoughts. When you catch yourself feeling a strong emotion, ask yourself: *What am I thinking right now?* or *Is this true?* If you catch yourself thinking something negative, you can say 'Stop!', and see if you can come up with a neutral thought replacement. It can also be helpful to write down your thoughts during this exercise.

Let's look at some common negative thoughts of hopelessness in grief and some suggestions on how you could reframe them.

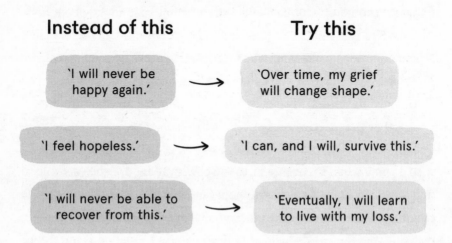

Instead of this

'I will never be happy again.'

'I feel hopeless.'

'I will never be able to recover from this.'

Try this

'Over time, my grief will change shape.'

'I can, and I will, survive this.'

'Eventually, I will learn to live with my loss.'

Im

When Mum died, it was almost impossible to feel any hope or optimism for the future. It felt like all the colour had drained out of my life. It was three months shy of my daughter's first birthday – a time that is supposed to be full of joy – and all I could think about was that my mum never got the chance to sing my daughter 'Happy Birthday' or write her a card. The thought of celebrating anything without her felt wrong.

I couldn't bear it when people would say to me, 'It doesn't get easier.' I was in so much pain that the thought of my grief not getting any easier to live with felt unbearable. I won't lie, they were right. But what I will tell you is that all those heavy emotions do become more manageable, and for me, that was a huge relief.

On the days when I felt hopeless, the best advice I was given was to take things minute by minute. Any time I found myself focusing on the future and all the things my mum would miss out on, I would bring myself back into the present moment. I would smell my daughter's baby scent and stroke her soft skin. If she was asleep, I would count things around the room – anything that would help get me out of my head.

When my daughter turned three and we celebrated her birthday, I took some time to reflect back on how I felt in the beginning. I was in a completely different headspace and although the day was still hard without my mum, I was also able to enjoy moments that I never thought I would again.

If you are feeling stuck in a dark hole of grief, strip back all your expectations. Start by taking things minute by minute, day by day, and hold onto one small but realistic expectation that something good is going to happen in the future and that you won't feel this level of pain forever. Cultivating hope and resilience after loss takes work, but no matter how hopeless you may be feeling right now, the colour will eventually make its way back into your life. I promise.

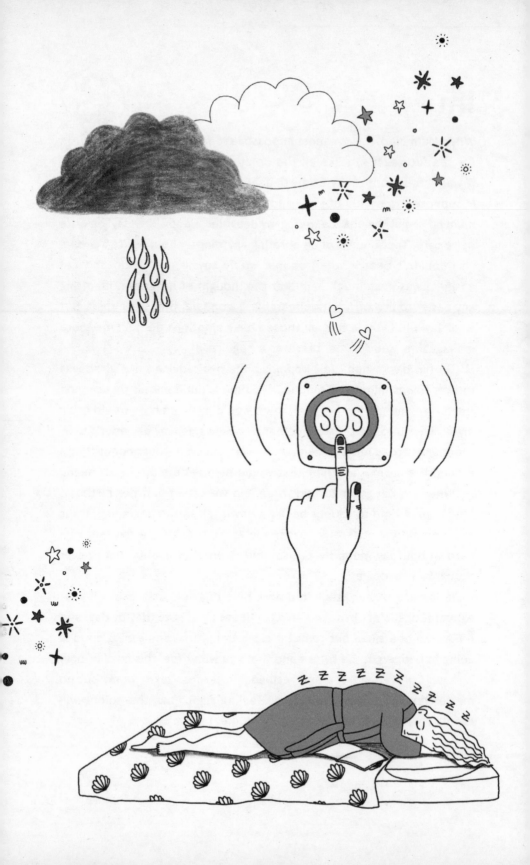

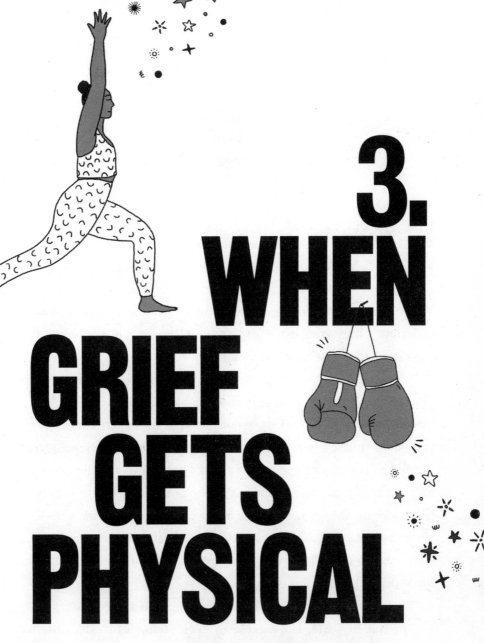

3.
WHEN GRIEF GETS PHYSICAL

Panic attacks,
exhaustion and
other fun stuff

YOUR BODY HURTS. YOU'VE GOT SCRAMBLED EGGS FOR BRAINS.

You're experiencing an array of physical symptoms and you're late-night googling: 'Does grief make you anxious?' and 'Is it normal to feel exhausted after loss?'. Sound familiar?

It's no secret that grief can mess with your emotions, but the physical symptoms of grief may come as a shock. For starters, grief is exhausting. We aren't talking about just your average tiredness. It's a can't-drag-yourself-out-of-bed level of fatigue, where putting one foot in front of the other seems almost impossible. You may also feel your loss so acutely that every bone in your body aches. Some days it's hard to muster up the energy to have a shower, and all you want to do is sleep. Yet when your head hits the pillow, your mind begins to race with anxious thoughts, trying to wrap itself around the fact that your loved one is gone.

There's a lot happening for you right now. It's no wonder you're feeling out of sorts, and unable to even string a bloody sentence together. Confronting your grief head-on, and 'taking each day as it comes', actually takes considerable work. Please remember: it's not you, it's *grief*. And although it may feel relentless, this slogfest of unpleasant symptoms will eventually subside.

SURVIVAL MODE: ACTIVATED

There is a very good explanation as to why grief takes such a toll on the body. The emotional stress you experience after a loss is perceived by the brain as a threat to survival, causing your brain to default to 'fight or flight' mode (aka survival mode). When this happens, the fear centre part of your brain starts to dominate. Your amygdala (a small part of your brain's limbic system, which is the part that regulates all those fun emotions we touched on in Chapter 2, along with scanning the environment for threats) acts as an alarm system. It screams that you're in danger, sending an SOS to your nervous system by flooding your body with stress hormones (cortisol and adrenaline).

While this response enables you to react quickly in life-threatening situations (thanks, evolution!), it can also trigger physiological reactions, including a pounding heart, rapid breathing, trembling and muscle tension. We spoke to Dr Lisa M. Shulman, a world-renowned neurologist and author of *Before and After Loss: A neurologist's perspective on loss, grief and our brain*. Dr Shulman explained that living in the mode of chronic stress can have a long-lasting impact on your brain function, respiratory system, digestive system, immune system, nervous system, heart function, sleep, libido and overall health and wellbeing. You know – all the fun stuff! She also said that the goal of the brain when you are experiencing emotional trauma is to keep you highly functional, so you can survive through difficult times.

Every time you are triggered by something after a loss (which we know can happen frequently), the alarm system activates. Living in survival mode is exhausting. All your internal resources are working on overdrive to keep you functioning, and this consistent and ongoing state of alarm can leave you feeling overwhelmed and anxious.

It's not only after a death that stress and survival mode might jump into action. It can also occur when you know death is imminent, or if you're caring for a loved one at the end of life. It is important to take care of yourself in the process (more on this in Chapter 4).

RELEASING STRESS FROM THE BODY

The good news is that there are ways to help you reduce your stress levels and start to heal your body and mind. Often when you're feeling stressed, exhausted and griefy, the last thing you want to do is peel yourself off the couch and hit up the gym. However, this is often the time when you could really benefit from getting your body moving. As little as 30 minutes of daily exercise has been scientifically proven to reduce stress and release endorphins, which are feel-good hormones. They can help to balance out the yucky stress hormones that are lingering in your body.

Another effective way to help ourselves cope after loss by releasing trauma and stress from our body is through breath-work. You've probably heard of the 'mind–body connection', the concept that our brains and bodies are intimately connected and influence one another. According to integrative somatic trauma therapist Rebecca Jax, it's common in grief to shut down and disconnect from the parts where you feel pain and anguish. This can keep you operating at a lower frequency where you might feel 'stuck', or constantly fatigued. Breath-work, Rebecca explains, is a powerful tool to create shifts in the brain and body, and release energetic and emotional blocks.

The importance of breathing is obvious, but we can easily forget how to breathe properly when we're operating in survival mode. Our breathing can become shallow, which exacerbates feelings of anxiety, causing us to feel even more out of control and in a state of panic. Deep breathing increases the supply of oxygen to your brain and stimulates the parasympathetic nervous system, which promotes a state of calm. It allows for healing on a cellular level and also breaks subconscious patterns, minimises feelings of dissociation and improves concentration and emotional regulation.

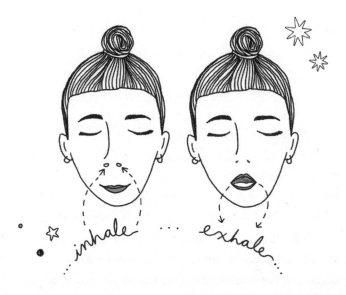

We love Rebecca's approach to healing, which is equal parts scientific and spiritual, so much so that we asked her to share with us a deep breathing exercise for you to try at home (see page 84). One of the critical aspects of working somatically, Rebecca says, is to prepare your mind and body for what's ahead. Before you jump into Rebecca's breath-work exercise, we want to highlight that it is an intense exercise designed to release trauma and stress from your body, and it may cause an emotional release. Breathing deeply takes work and may not feel relaxing, and it's important to take the breaths at your own pace. Rebecca suggests you find a comfy space in your home and play some calming music. It's a good idea to have a glass of water, tissues and a blanket nearby, as well as a journal to write about your experience afterwards.

A DEEP-BREATHING EXERCISE

by Rebecca Jax

1. Find a comfortable position sitting or lying down. Keep your arms and legs uncrossed, with your palms facing up.
2. Begin to inhale slowly through your nose, allowing your belly to rise as your diaphragm fills up with air.
3. Exhale through your mouth, making the exhale long (as if you are pushing energy away from your body with the breath). You may begin to feel a tingling sensation in your fingers and toes.
4. Continue for 20 breaths in total, with no pause in between. It is a conscious connected breath, an infinite breath with no beginning and no end.
5. Once you have done 20 breaths, exhale and then hold your breath on empty lungs for 20 seconds.
6. Repeat this for three rounds, completing 20 deep diaphragmatic breaths, followed by a 20-second breath-hold for each round.
7. Move as you activate the parts of your body where you are holding a lot of tension. Allow your body to move in whatever way feels comfortable. You could try rocking your hips, rolling your shoulders back, and stretching your neck.

When you have completed the three rounds of breath-work, grab your journal and answer the following questions.

*   *Where am I holding tension and stress in my body?*
*   *What emotion am I resisting the most?*
*   *What can I let go of today?*

Please remember, there's no one right approach to healing or releasing trauma, and breath-work may not be for everyone. It can be helpful to experiment with different tools when processing your loss.

Katharina's experience with stress and exhaustion

'My mum died six months after a cancer diagnosis, in June 2021. She and I were very close, she was my confidante and I miss her terribly. What completely surprised me, though, was the level of physical exhaustion I was experiencing. Before Mum's death, I was very active. I went to the gym, met with friends and was always full of energy – I lived life to the fullest. A whole weekend on the couch, watching movies and doing nothing? Not for me! I had things to do and people to meet. However, after Mum's death, I couldn't do that anymore. I just about managed to go to work and do the bare necessities. On the weekends, I felt deeply exhausted and tired and just wanted to be left alone, preferably under a blanket with →

◁ some tea. Where did all my energy go? Sure, I was sad and angry and grieving, but why did my body feel like I had just run a marathon, when I was living my normal day-to-day life? It felt very isolating and depleting.'

What helped

'Learning that extreme emotional stress can manifest physically has helped me to better look after myself and allow my body to rest. I take things easy and I've adjusted my expectations of what I can do.'

Jacqueline's experience with stress and exhaustion

'I have never experienced grief like the loss of my husband to suicide. He was incredibly intelligent and a loving partner and father. We were together for over two decades and married for almost 14 years. Exhaustion is something I have felt since the day he died. It can feel all-consuming and paralysing. There are layers of guilt, stress and shame that accompany exhaustion, because I feel silly to be so tired from attending a meeting or going to the grocery store. But that's what it feels like – everything takes so much more mental and physical energy to complete than before he died.

'I like to imagine exhaustion as a wave. Depending on how I'm feeling, that helps me figure out if I want to ride the wave by doing something active, or by seeking some form of rest. I have found that sometimes I need to manage the exhaustion by finding a project/task or physical activity to help me get through it. The hardest thing to do to deal with exhaustion has been to rest, both physically and emotionally, when my body needs it.'

What helped

'Adding things to my calendar like "nap" reminds me what my body and broken heart need that day to make it easier to set aside the "should be doing" things. Giving myself permission to stay in bed and be sad, or whatever it is that feels right for me at that time, helps me be more present and patient with my children, friends and family. This can also mean setting boundaries with those around me, prioritising my mental and physical health. I resist judgement on the days where I need to move more slowly and look inwards, and embrace the days where I feel more open to engaging with the world around me.'

GRIEF AND LACK OF SLEEP

Another outcome of prolonged stress in grief is unrelenting tiredness. No, scrap that – it's extreme full-body exhaustion that feels utterly debilitating. Your eyeballs are tired from crying and your heart feels tired from hurting. No amount of sleep seems to restore your energy. It's yet another long-lasting symptom on the big old list of 'Griefy things nobody warned us about'. It's a type of tiredness that is hard to shake, even if you're getting early nights and doing all the right things to look after yourself.

No surprises on this one – according to a 2010 study by the University of Pittsburgh School of Medicine, sleep disturbances are very common among the bereaved. You might be having nightmares or dreaming about your person, which leads to a bad sleep. Or, you could be putting off going to bed and instead staying up until the early hours – something that might feel good in the moment, but which can wreak havoc on your sleep cycle. Falling asleep can be difficult, too, as distressing and griefy thoughts from the day can flood in, keeping you awake. And even if you do fall asleep, you might wake up throughout the night. All in all, sleep can be hard to come by in grief, and you might wake up feeling like you've run a marathon, rather than restored your energy. It can become a bit of a cycle: grief causes sleep disturbances, and sleep disturbances can exacerbate feelings of grief. What a predicament.

Sleep improves memory retention and recall, so when you're deprived of it, both these areas can be impacted. It plays a big role in the consolidation of memories (where your brain files them away for long-term use), but when you're lacking sleep, your brain's neurons are overworked and you can't coordinate information properly. Focus, attention and vigilance drift, making it more difficult to receive and retain information.

Psychologist Tamara's view on coping with stress

Grief is associated with feelings of hopelessness, anxiety and stress, and all of these feelings have very real corresponding physical changes.

Grief is something you have to go through – there is no way to avoid it, ignore it or control it. So when you have a private moment, allow yourself to cry. Research shows that tears release important chemicals associated with relief and positive emotions. Understand that crying is, in fact, healing. It's acknowledging the depth of your loss. Remind yourself that it's normal to not be okay, and that your mood may change from hour to hour and even minute by minute.

When functioning in survival mode, it can be helpful to focus on the simple. Small goals are important and they need to be recognised as achievement. Just eating counts. Just showering is a success. When your pain is all-encompassing, just being able to do the smallest thing is, in fact, an achievement – remind yourself of that. Set a routine and build on it. Our bodies feel comfort in predictability, and stress responses reduce with increasing stimuli or with achievement.

Routine can provide comfort and knowledge that you can continue and function despite a life-changing loss. This is your time to take the best possible care of yourself.

Sal

I've always been a heavy sleeper. After Mum died, I was exhausted but my body was running on adrenaline, so I felt wired all the time. As soon as my head touched the pillow at night, I felt overcome with grief. I'd lie there and sob, feeling a deep ache in my chest. After a busy day, my mind wasn't consumed with all of the things I had to get done – finally, I was still and had space to process my emotions. I'd lie awake and think about my mum, about how I was going to get through this, about the pain – all of it.

During those months I decided that if sleep was hard to come by, I at least needed to give my body a chance to rest, so I could tackle the next day. I started to implement a simple rest routine each night to help me wind down before bed and decompress, so I wouldn't feel as stressed. I wanted to give myself the best chance of feeling calm. I powered down all devices, switched my phone to flight mode, made myself a chamomile tea and put on a sleep mask to block out any light. They're pretty simple things, really, but they made a genuine difference in helping me get into the right frame of mind, and relax, before trying to get some sleep. On the nights when my mind was whirring with griefy thoughts, I noticed that I felt more able to relax and process things.

Sal's 'rest and reset' bedtime checklist

When you're grieving, you don't have a lot of mental energy to spend. Rather than trying to implement a fancy bedtime routine, making a few tweaks to your 'sleep hygiene' might help you get a better night's rest. We conducted a short poll within our Instagram community, and 87 per cent of members reported that they, too, suffer from a lack of sleep after loss.

Here's a bedtime checklist I put together to help you get started (it's best to pick one or two things, rather than try to do it all).

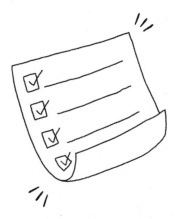

* Make sure your room is dark and at a comfortable, cool temperature.
* Limit napping in the day if you can.
* Allow yourself a wind-down window of 30 minutes before bedtime to decompress.
* Avoid looking at any screens for at least 30 minutes before bedtime (your phone, TV, tablet and laptop). If you do need to look at a screen, try using a blue light filter, which can help increase the sleep-promoting hormone, melatonin.
* If practical, turn your phone to 'do not disturb' mode.
* If your mind is racing, do a brain dump before bed and write down everything that's in your head. This can help to clear your thoughts.
* Steer clear of any caffeine or sugary foods in the evenings.
* Magnesium supplements play a role in calming your nervous system, which can promote sleep. Try taking magnesium powder an hour before bed.
* Try a relaxation technique, such as a guided meditation.

If your sleep isn't improving, another option is to see a psychologist about cognitive behavioural therapy (CBT) for insomnia.

What our community said about . . .

GRIEF AND SLEEP

'I have only been getting about four to five hours of sleep a night and I'm exhausted.'

'I wake up and – *BANG* – I remember they're gone again, and I can't get back to sleep.'

'My sleep is so broken. I keep having nightmares and waking up in a panic.'

'I find it hard to switch off my brain and I have lots of awful dreams.'

'I wake up every night with racing thoughts and a pounding heartbeat.'

'I wake up in the middle of the night thinking about his accident.'

'I keep having the same recurring nightmares and find it difficult to get back to sleep.'

'As soon as I try to go to sleep, I start over-analysing everything in detail.'

GRIEF BRAIN

Have you heard of 'baby brain'? It's the term used to describe the mental fog, absent-mindedness, memory problems and poor concentration experienced by mothers of newborns. 'Grief brain', also known as 'grief brain fog' or 'griever's fog', is similar. Have you been feeling foggy and forgetful or like your brain's gone *KAPUT*? You may even be using up a lot of brain juice just attempting to read this book. Grief brain is very real, and a lot of people don't even realise that it's an actual thing.

Dr Lisa M. Shulman conducted research on how grief impacts the brain after her husband died from cancer and disorientation became a big issue for her. Even though she was an experienced neurologist, the way grief impacted her brain surprised her, so she started to dig deeper. Through her research, she came up with a theory on why people feel mentally foggy after a loss. Basically, the stress response plays a big role in our brain's function (or, more accurately, dysfunction). She says that a key part to understanding what is going on in the brain is to realise that the brain rewires itself after loss. Chronic stress activates neuroplasticity and it also weakens nerve growth, resulting in memory impairment and increased fear. These weakened neural connections, plus a whole host of other psychological defence mechanisms, impact the different 'cognitive domains'. These domains are memory, executive function, attention, word fluency and speed of information processing. Dr Shulman explained that 'neurons that fire together, wire together', which essentially means that if chronic stress causes a circuit of anxiety and fear to repeatedly fire away in the brain, it becomes a default setting. The more it's reinforced, the more it's getting hard wired, which explains why brain fog can linger for ages after loss. If things don't make much sense or you're forgetful and confused, understand that it does not mean that there's anything fundamentally wrong with you – it's grief.

RIGHT NOW,

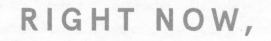

OF ANY EXPECTATIONS OF YOURSELF.

YOU DON'T HAVE TO HAVE IT ALL FIGURED OUT.

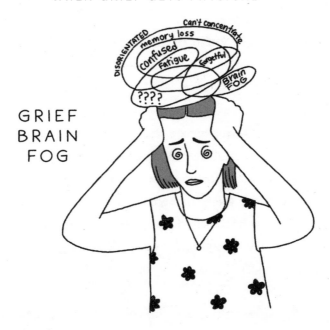

GRIEF
BRAIN
FOG

If you're struggling with grief brain fog in your day-to-day life, here are some suggestions that might help.

- Set reminders on your phone and in your calendar to keep on top of deadlines or appointments. Try setting them for a day before the deadline/event, then a few hours before, then an hour before.
- Make lists of everything you need to get done. It can be helpful to have a list stuck somewhere central, such as your fridge, so you can easily see it and add to it.
- Take lots of notes! In fact, make sticky notes your best friend. When you think of something to do, write it on one and stick it somewhere obvious.
- Try to limit distractions if you're having trouble concentrating at work.
- Email yourself when you have a thought or remember something. That way, when you check your inbox, you can diarise it or action it when you're ready.

Journalling to alleviate brain fog

According to Dr Shulman, it is possible to combat brain fog and restore your brain's cognitive function. She suggests that journalling can act as a mindfulness and relaxation practice and help promote feelings of calmness, which in turn alleviate stress and encourage clarity. It gives you an outlet to let out all the whirring thoughts and feelings that you may be stuffing down inside you. Putting pen to paper can allow you to separate some of the griefy thoughts in your head and dig a little bit deeper into how you're really feeling. Also, when you're writing in a journal, you can let rip and really write for you and you only. There's power in opening up, because you don't need to censor any of your thoughts or hold anything back.

Expressing yourself through the act of writing is key to working through stress and traumatic events. You might choose to let loose and write pages, or maybe only a few sentences, or jot down a random thought or memory. Whatever comes into your mind at the time, just write it down. Don't overthink it or put pressure on yourself to do it every day. Think of journalling as a griefy brain dump, because the words might come thick and fast, and make no sense when you re-read them, but it feels better once you've released them onto the page.

Set aside some time to write about what's going on for you. Find a calm and relaxing space where you can really sink into the practice. There's no pressure to come up with anything grand, just write what you are feeling at this very moment. If that seems like too much, maybe you might find comfort in writing down some of your favourite memories of your person.

Farhan's experience with 'grief brain and body'

'Grief, for me, impacts more than my brain – I feel like I have a "grief body". Some days I'm incapacitated physically and mentally. I lie on the couch, eyes closed and exhausted. I can't think, I can't move and I can't sleep. I feel a dense fog around my head and my body feels like it's covered in thick, dark tar. Every move requires contemplation and effort. I literally feel like I am the walking dead.

'Then there are days where I am more mentally impacted and that presents with forgetfulness, such as walking into a room and not remembering why I went there. I misplace things a lot, I forget the names of places and people that normally roll off my tongue. As I speak or write, I forget words and my thoughts mid-sentence. I also forget where I parked my car and often have to circle multiple times before finding my spot.'

What helped

'I begin each morning with meditation. Some days I can focus and get a deeper connection in my practice, but there are days when I'm simply going through the motions. I also make a list of everything I have to do each day. Once it's down on paper, I simply work through my list. I don't put pressure on myself to complete everything that's on there. I try to be gentle with myself. A regular workout at the gym helps me get into my body and clears my mind. The most important thing I've learned is to exercise self-compassion.'

What our community said about . . .

GRIEF BRAIN

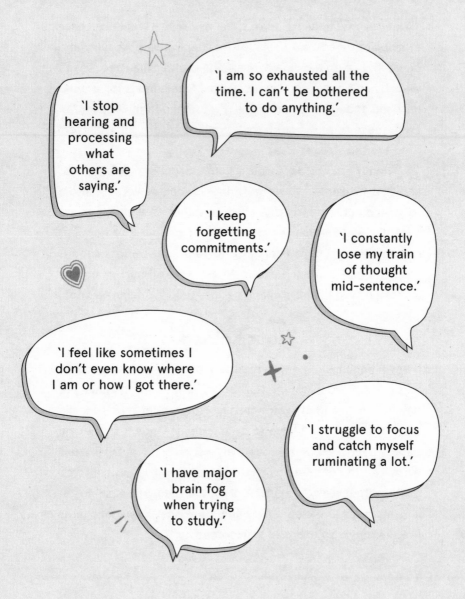

'I stop hearing and processing what others are saying.'

'I am so exhausted all the time. I can't be bothered to do anything.'

'I keep forgetting commitments.'

'I constantly lose my train of thought mid-sentence.'

'I feel like sometimes I don't even know where I am or how I got there.'

'I struggle to focus and catch myself ruminating a lot.'

'I have major brain fog when trying to study.'

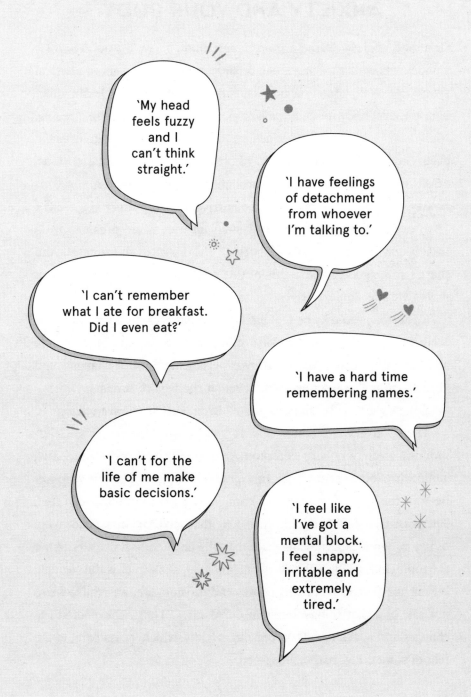

ANXIETY AND YOUR BODY

Grief and anxiety. Name a more iconic duo . . . we'll wait. You may wonder why we are talking about anxiety in a chapter all about physical symptoms. Well, anxiety is not just experienced mentally. It can affect your physical body in many ways, too, especially when you're grieving. No wonder – because you're dealing with one of life's most stressful events and you're experiencing a whole range of unpleasant emotions. Stress hormones are surging through your body. Insomnia is your new best friend. Your brain has been triggered to protect you from a (non-existent) physical threat. There's an unrealistic pressure from society for you to be 'back to normal' shortly after the funeral. And there's still a good-sized chunk of this book to go, with a multitude of ways that grief impacts your life.

Right now, you may be feeling like grief has impacted your sense of security and safety, and the world suddenly feels like an unpredictable and unfamiliar place. You're likely experiencing a lot of changes, and change can feel really unsettling, even at the best of times.

What's there to be anxious about? Errrr. Just about *everything*!

The good news is (once again!): you're not alone in this. Grief-induced anxiety is very common. In fact, we both experienced it, along with 95 per cent of our Instagram community. Anyone who has been in the grip of anxiety will know how all-consuming it can feel. Therapist Claire Bidwell Smith told us that anxiety impacts so many of her patients experiencing grief that she decided to write a book on the topic. In *Anxiety: The missing stage of grief*, she explains that when a big change (such as a death) comes and disrupts life, we realise we're not safe and that things aren't in our control. These unexpected life changes and a lack of safety feed our anxiety, which, at its core, is the fear of something, real or imagined.

Anxiety is intrinsically linked to our physiology, Claire explains. You might have physical pain or sensations that generate a fear-based thought or memory, or you might have a fear-based thought that generates a physical sensation. According to Claire, what sets grief-related anxiety apart from generalised anxiety is that there is a very specific trigger for fear-based thoughts, which stems from the experience of loss. Your body is designed to react to fear and, after experiencing loss, she says, many of the fears that run through your mind are perceived as more of a threat than before the loss. Someone has died, making death very real, so that inevitability is now more prominent for you in your life.

Claire says that when you experience fear-based thoughts about your person's death, your own mortality or someone else's, your body and mind are actually reacting in a stronger way than before you experienced loss firsthand. Grieving people, she explains, can feel worried about their own health or the safety of other loved ones without even realising that what they are experiencing is anxiety, or that it's even related to their grief. That's why your anxiety might be stronger in relation to certain things than it was prior to your loss.

GRIEF TIP

Worrying can become addictive. When we worry too much, it creates a cycle that's difficult to break. You may find that your anxious thoughts become a comfort blanket, keeping you 'prepared' just in case something else goes wrong. However, it's important to recognise the worrying thoughts and try to shift the focus. The key is to not get wrapped up in them, and instead, think of something positive. Other things that can help when you feel your thoughts starting to spiral are changing your environment, phoning a friend, or taking a few slow, deep breaths.

Im

At the age of 17, I was diagnosed with generalised anxiety disorder (GAD). I know what it feels like to live in a constant state of impending doom, and to worry incessantly over things that are beyond your control. I've had CT scans and rushed myself to hospital, convinced that I was dying, only to be told I was having a panic attack. I could not comprehend how something that's essentially mental can feel so damn physical and frightening. Over the years, I accepted my diagnosis, and, through lots of therapy, have learned ways to manage my anxiety. I hadn't experienced a panic attack for a long time.

When Mum died, my anxiety went to town. All my hard mental-work started unravelling and I was right back in the shoes of 17-year-old anxious me. Only this time, I had real cause for concern. Death was all of a sudden very real for me.

I was standing at the supermarket check-out, about to go and pick up my daughter from day care. It was one of those average griefy days – the ones where you aren't uncontrollably sobbing and grief feels somewhat manageable. Well, that was until my heart started pounding out of my chest. My hands went clammy and tingly. My body was trembling. I felt completely disconnected from everything around me, and I was convinced it was my time to go. *Here we go again. This ain't my first rodeo,* I thought. Although on this occasion, it felt much, much worse. Grief-induced anxiety is on another level.

Having had previous experience with anxiety, I was pulling out all the stops – I focused on taking slow, deep breaths and repeatedly told myself, *You're not going crazy. You're not going to die.* Luckily, the symptoms started to subside after a few minutes, but the aftermath lingered in my system, and I felt exhausted, shaky and on edge for days.

It's crucial to familiarise yourself with the symptoms of a panic attack in case you do experience one. Arming yourself with the knowledge of what's happening to you physically can help you remain calm in the moment, and allow you to talk yourself down from *I'm dying*, to *I'm grieving and living in survival mode and my constant worry has tricked my body into thinking there is a physical threat.*

After someone dies, you may wonder, *Who's next?* Experiencing intense fear that you, or everyone around you, are no longer safe, is very normal and common. Much like grief, anxiety isn't something that will disappear entirely, but you can learn to accept it as part of you. It's important to put practices into place to keep on top of your mental health, especially when coping with loss.

If you do struggle with anxiety, check out @anxietyjosh on Instagram. Joshua Fletcher is an anxiety therapist and the co-author of *Untangle Your Anxiety: A guide to overcoming an anxiety disorder by two people who have been through it.* His content was game-changing for me!

Signs of a panic attack

- ☐ RESTLESSNESS
- ☐ RACING THOUGHTS
- ☐ DIZZINESS
- ☐ FEELING FAINT
- ☐ FEELING DISORIENTED
- ☐ FEAR OF LOSING CONTROL
- ☐ INCREASED HEART RATE
- ☐ LOSS OF APPETITE
- ☐ SWEATING
- ☐ CHILLS OR HOT FLUSHES
- ☐ TREMBLING, TINGLING OR FEELING NUMB
- ☐ SHORTNESS OF BREATH
- ☐ UPSET STOMACH OR NAUSEA
- ☐ JELLY LEGS
- ☐ DRY MOUTH
- ☐ TIGHTNESS IN CHEST/CHEST PAIN

Try the '5-4-3-2-1' method

A popular tool for helping to ease anxiety is practising what is called the '5-4-3-2-1' technique to ground and calm yourself when feeling upset, anxious or untethered.

Here's how to do it:

5 Look for five things you can see. Maybe it's something on your desk, through the window, or something you are wearing.

4 Become aware of four things you can touch. Perhaps it's a pen, your laptop or the fabric of your clothes.

3 Acknowledge three things you can hear. It could be a noise in the distance, or the sound of your breath.

2 Take note of two things you can smell. It could be a cup of coffee, or your colleague's perfume.

1 Be aware of one thing you can taste. If you can't taste anything, name a taste that you like instead.

Meditation to help ease anxiety

When anxiety feels all-consuming, a consistent meditation practice can help to reduce stress and calm your nervous system. Meditation helps you regulate your emotions and learn body awareness so that you can become more attuned to the physical sensations you are experiencing and start to chill out. There are a few ways that you can use meditation to manage anxiety and stress. A good place to start when your body is reacting to anxiety is a meditation known as a 'body scan'. You can practise this either lying down, sitting with your feet flat on the floor or standing up. Close your eyes and mentally scan your body, inch by inch, from head to toe. Bring your awareness to your breath by taking slow, deep breaths, in through your nose and out through your mouth. Starting at the top of your head, relax your muscles and let go of any tension in your face. Continue this through your torso, arms, hands, abdomen, legs and all the way down to your toes. Spend a little longer focused on the areas where you feel discomfort, by breathing slowly into those places. Try this for three minutes. This is also a great exercise to practise if you are having trouble falling asleep.

Another meditation exercise you could try is what's called a 'walking meditation' or 'mindful walking', where you focus on putting one foot in front of the other, step by step, paying attention to the sensation of your feet coming into contact with the ground. As you start to walk, notice how your body feels. Does it feel heavy or light? This exercise can be done anywhere and is a really good way to get your body moving while bringing you back to the present moment, connecting with nature and your surroundings.

If you're struggling to concentrate when doing your own meditation, there are some wonderful apps available that have a whole range of guided meditation practices you could try, including Headspace, Insight Timer, Calm and Smiling Mind.

Another effective tool to ease feelings of anxiety is repeating simple, calming mantras (out loud or in your head – whatever is comfortable for you). Affirmations can help override negative or worrisome thoughts and replace them with more positive ones. Here are some of our favourites:

'I am safe. I am calm.'
'This too shall pass.'
'This feeling is only temporary.'
'I won't feel this way forever.'

What our community said about . . .

WHAT HELPS THEM WHEN FEELING ANXIOUS

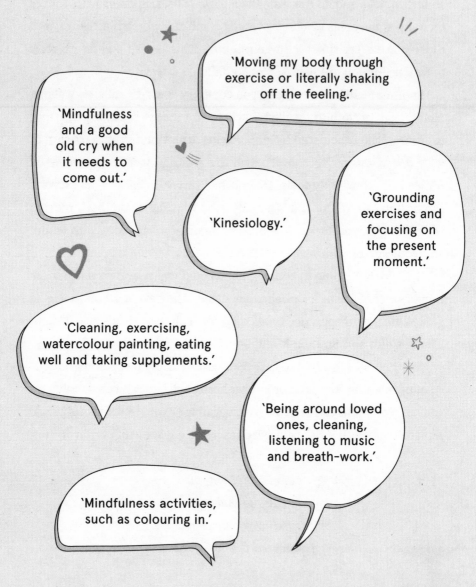

'Moving my body through exercise or literally shaking off the feeling.'

'Mindfulness and a good old cry when it needs to come out.'

'Kinesiology.'

'Grounding exercises and focusing on the present moment.'

'Cleaning, exercising, watercolour painting, eating well and taking supplements.'

'Being around loved ones, cleaning, listening to music and breath-work.'

'Mindfulness activities, such as colouring in.'

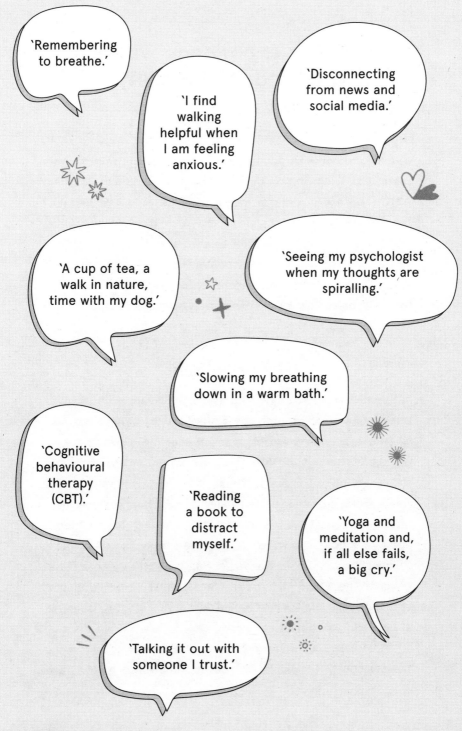

Tilly's experience with grief-induced anxiety

'My dad died in March 2017. Shortly before that, my dear mum was diagnosed with dementia and then, over the next few years, with two different types of cancer. She died in October 2020. The experience of losing both parents and being a carer, and the trauma of watching my mum die, left me feeling anxious. I've always been familiar with anxiety, but this was a whole new ball game. It was constant, all-encompassing and extremely overwhelming. I experienced violent nightmares, terrifying panic attacks and exhaustion from being in a constant state of "fight or flight".'

What helped

'Alternative therapies have helped me, especially acupuncture. During one appointment, my acupuncturist suggested that when overwhelming anxiety washed over me, I should try to physically shake it off, like an animal would in the wild, and fully exert myself – punch the air (hard!) for one minute, do fierce star jumps and shake my entire body, even my face. Yes, I felt weird, but it really worked to shift the fear. My boyfriend and I have been known to do it on the side of the road when things got too much – if I was crying, or getting into a state of panic, he would just shout, "Star jumps!" It would nearly always change the scene from an ugly crying mess to laughing at how silly we looked.

'A trick I've also learned from my therapist is that when anxiety comes knocking, I sit down somewhere quiet, start doing some breathing exercises and find my happy place. The place can be real or imaginary, but I really picture it, immersing myself in it. My happy place is a place in India I want to revisit. I put on my headphones with nature sounds playing and I imagine myself sitting there, listening to the sea, smelling the dhal cooking for lunch and the incense wafting past my nose, feeling the sun on my face. It helps everything feel less scary and brings me back to myself.'

Anxiety and alcohol

We've touched on how survival mode can disrupt the balance of chemicals and processes in your brain. Well, so does alcohol. Grief already feels like a really bad, constant hangover; sprinkle a couple of spicy margs in there and it's a recipe for 'hang-xiety', which is a hangover and anxiety all rolled into one very unpleasant feeling from hell. Turning to booze after a loss can be a coping mechanism for some, but even having as little as one or two alcoholic drinks when you're grieving can leave you feeling highly anxious and foggier than ever in the following days.

We spoke with anxiety expert, Claire Bidwell Smith, about why booze makes our anxiety so much worse. She said that while it might make you feel a bit looser emotionally at first, when it leaves your system you can have fluctuating chemicals and hormones, which can make you feel terrible. Alcohol might feel like a friend at first, Claire says, but it doesn't help you in the long run. It acts as a chemical depressant, affecting your thoughts and feelings, which can then have a negative impact on your overall mental health and wellbeing. If you have been turning to alcohol as a bit of a suppressant, why not try cutting back a bit and seeing how you feel? A clearer mind and less anxiety may be exactly what you need right now.

WHEN YOUR LOSS IS TRAUMATIC

When you experience a loss that was sudden, unexpected and/or violent in nature, such as homicide, suicide, an accident or natural disaster, the trauma response can be so severe that it can complicate the natural grief process.

The shock and unexpected nature of your loss can trigger overwhelming amounts of stress and preoccupying thoughts, which can significantly impact your day-to-day life. According to author, psychotherapist and trauma specialist Britt Frank, a traumatic loss can put you on a loop where you continuously experience the shock of the event, making it nearly impossible to grieve. You may feel like the world around you is unsafe and unpredictable, leading to increased feelings of fear and anxiety, making it exponentially harder to cope.

Much like grief, everyone responds to traumatic loss differently, but here are some of the ways it can show up:

- intrusive thoughts, images and flashbacks
- sleep disturbances or nightmares
- anxiety or panic attacks
- avoiding reminders that link you to the event (such as people, places, objects and activities)
- feeling detached from yourself or the world around you
- difficulty concentrating
- ruminating thoughts
- hypervigilance and being easily startled.

In *The Body Keeps the Score: Brain, mind, and body in the healing of trauma*, world-leading expert on trauma Dr Bessel van der Kolk explains that the lives of many trauma survivors come to revolve around bracing against, and neutralising, unwanted sensory experiences, such as shock.

Because trauma can become stored inside the body, when people are chronically angry or scared, constant muscle tension (a symptom of attempting to cope with trauma) can show up as back pain, migraine headaches and other forms of chronic pain. For many trauma survivors, he explains, it can be difficult to relax and feel fully safe in their body, and so one of the most effective alternative therapies for releasing trauma from your body is practising yoga. It focuses your attention on your breathing and bodily sensations. You begin to notice the connection between your emotions and your body and, in turn, noticing what you are feeling helps with emotional regulation. What's more, Dr van der Kolk explains, trauma can make you feel stuck in a state of fear, but yoga teaches you that emotions come and go. Over time, it might help your emotions feel more manageable, rather than being hijacked by them.

It's nearly impossible to grieve when your nervous system is constantly primed for threat. If you're experiencing any of the symptoms we've mentioned, you may want to seek some extra support by speaking to a therapist who specialises in traumatic grief. The goal of therapy is never to 'get over' what happened. The goal of therapy is to deactivate the inner alarm system so you can observe your thoughts and safely access your emotions and bodily sensations related to the loss.

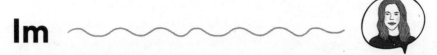

Im

Suicide is an unbelievably traumatic and catastrophic way to lose someone you love. There are so many unanswered questions, as it goes against the grain of one of the most basic human instincts: to survive. For me, it was utterly incomprehensible how my mum could have taken her own life. On top of this, the violent nature of my mum's death, and the complex circumstances surrounding it, added many complicated layers of trauma to my loss that I had to (and still have to) process and work through every single day.

For about ten months, I felt mentally stuck at the time and place of my mum's death, unable to move past it or function as well as I normally could. I was frightened to be alone. I struggled to sleep. I was afraid to shut my eyes because whenever I did, I would experience intrusive thoughts and images. I'd wake up frequently in the night and early hours of the morning, panicking. I'd spend my days ruminating and replaying all the details on a loop, trying to make sense of what had happened. You know when you have a nightmare, and you wake up and realise it was just a bad dream and you feel a sense of relief wash over you? I was waking up and my reality *was* the nightmare.

Therapy was a non-negotiable for me. I knew I needed extra support to help me cope and work through my trauma. I saw my GP almost immediately and got put on a mental health plan. I was seeing someone who specialises in bereavement by suicide as well as a psychotherapist and a forensic psychologist. I had therapy around the clock and found it incredibly helpful in processing my complicated thoughts and emotions.

On top of therapy, I took a holistic approach to healing and got regular acupuncture and kinesiology, practised breath-work and, even on days when I had no energy, I made sure I did at least 30 minutes of exercise. What's also helped me is falling asleep listening to guided meditation every night. My head was a horrible place to be, and my thoughts were too much to bear. I needed a distraction, and I found that listening to a soothing voice and calming music, and taking slow, deep breaths, really helps. Although it may not feel like it right now, with consistent and regular practices in place, it is possible to go beyond just surviving after experiencing a traumatic loss.

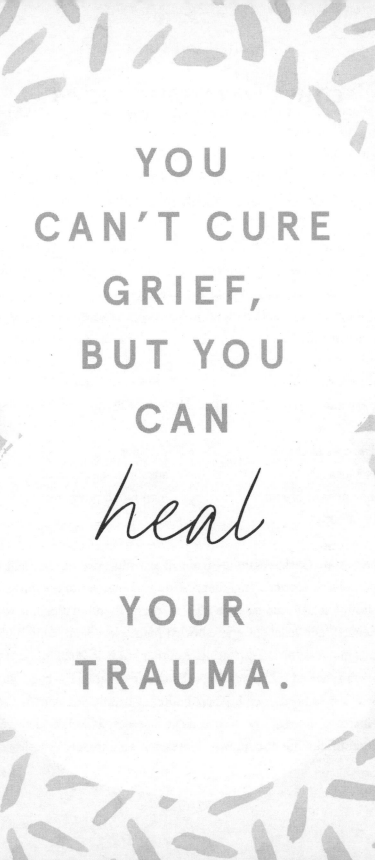

YOU CAN'T CURE GRIEF, BUT YOU CAN *heal* YOUR TRAUMA.

OTHER WAYS GRIEF SHOWS UP IN YOUR BODY

All the topics we've touched on – stress, exhaustion, sleep disturbances, brain fog and anxiety – are some of the ways that you might feel your body is battling with grief on a daily basis. But they aren't the only ways that grief can show up physically. The stress of grief can impact your appetite and weight. Some people undereat, some overeat, and some feel nauseous or experience digestive issues. Cramps, tremors, headaches, body aches, skin issues and cardiovascular issues are just a few of the many physical symptoms that people can experience. Here are some others:

- migraines
- tense jaw
- chest pains
- tightness in throat
- hair loss
- shortness of breath
- dry mouth
- hormonal changes
- loss of libido
- weakness
- dizziness
- autoimmune disorders
- high blood pressure.

Researcher Dr Chris Fagundes from Rice University in the US has studied the link between grief, depression and changes to the immune and cardiovascular systems. In a 2019 study, he found that people who experienced high levels of grief showed higher levels of the immune system's markers for inflammation. Another study in 2020 found that people who showed high psychological measures of grief also had higher levels of stress hormones in their bodies. Chronic stress can, over time, increase the risk of cardiovascular diseases, as well as diabetes, cancer, autoimmune conditions, depression and anxiety. The lesson here is that it's really important to take care of your physical health when you're deep in grief.

You know your body better than anyone else, so if you are experiencing any physical symptoms that you are at all concerned about, write them down in as much detail as you can and take your concerns to your GP to discuss.

Sal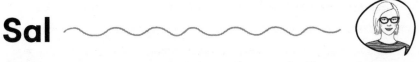

A few months before Mum died, I was diagnosed with an autoimmune disease. It was in the very early stages, so it was manageable. A week before Mum died, I had some blood tests done as part of a regular check-up. My levels were fine, and everything was under control.

A couple of months after Mum died, I had more blood tests and discovered that, in the space of eight weeks, the disease had significantly progressed and I needed to increase my dose of medication. My doctor explained that it was highly likely that the stress of grief had impacted my immune health, causing the disease to progress. Looking back at the initial months after Mum's death, I was under a lot of stress and I was feeling anxious and exhausted (not to mention grieving!). It made sense that my health had been impacted.

Robert's experience with emotional eating

'My wife was diagnosed with cancer in 2016 and I became her carer for the last 18 months of her life. I was very focused on looking after her and taking care of my young son's needs, and was so busy that I neglected my own needs. Instead of eating well, I just grabbed something quick to eat when I had a spare moment. Unsurprisingly, during that period I lost weight.

'Following my wife's death, my relationship with food began to change. In the evenings after I'd put my son to bed, I began to emotionally eat – in part because of boredom and loneliness, but also because it gave me a tiny moment of pleasure and comfort, amidst the pain of grief. Gradually I put on 32 kilograms. I was aware that I was putting on weight but my low self-worth and apathy at that time in my grief meant I didn't do anything about it.'

What helped

'The turning point was when I had a health scare that required surgery and was simultaneously diagnosed with hypertension. I realised that I needed to take my health seriously because I was my son's sole remaining parent. That drive helped me to make some dietary and lifestyle changes that have now helped me lose almost 41 kilograms.'

Helen's experience with the physical symptoms of grief

'My wonderful dad, Ian, died of COVID-19 on 12 April 2020. He was admitted to hospital on the day that our first national lockdown was announced in the UK, and remained in ICU for three weeks until no more could be done.

'I had always been fortunate enough to be fit and healthy, but after Dad died I started experiencing a variety of physical ailments. I developed acne on my face, followed by eczema flares on my eyelids. I then started experiencing debilitating dizziness and extreme pain in my lower back, which at the time I put down to the result of a more sedentary lifestyle from being in lockdown. I was also suffering from chronic fatigue but, again, blamed this on the fact that I was grieving, living in lockdown and furloughed from work.

'When it got to the point that I was being forced to crawl on the floor due to the immense pain I was experiencing and I was waking up in the middle of the night in tears from the agony, I knew I had to see a doctor. I ended up being diagnosed with a condition called ankylosing spondylitis, which is an inflammatory form of arthritis that mainly affects the spine. It is commonly associated with Crohn's disease, which I then ended up being diagnosed with, having previously put my bowel issues down to the fact I was stressed. Both of these autoimmune conditions are incurable, so having to learn to live with them has been a big adjustment, not only physically, but mentally, too.' →

What helped

'Though I always knew that grief could affect your physical health, I underestimated the scale on which this could happen. I've learned that physical aspects can last as long as your grief: forever. Listening to my body and trusting that I know it best has been key to coping. Rest and limiting stress are a necessity now because if I overdo it, my conditions will flare. My advice is to prioritise self-care, don't feel guilty for taking a break and, if something doesn't feel right, always seek medical advice as you can never underestimate the extent to which grief can manifest physically.'

SHOWING YOUR BODY SOME KINDNESS

Exercising self-compassion can be so important when you're wading through the physical symptoms of grief. In her book, *Self-compassion: The proven power of being kind to yourself*, Dr Kristen Neff identifies that there are three core components to practising self-compassion: self-kindness, common humanity and mindfulness. Dr Neff explains that it's important to give yourself the same caring support you'd give to a good friend, and this is especially true when you're grieving. We can be so hard on ourselves and set unrealistic expectations (as we discussed in Chapter 1). We need to show ourselves a little kindness and understand that what we're going through is really tough. Grief is messy and enormously confusing. You may not be able to function in the same capacity that you did pre-grief, and that's okay. There is a lot going on for you emotionally and physically. As cheesy as it may sound, it's important to show yourself a lot of love and kindness during this time – because you bloody well deserve it.

Here are our go-to ways to show ourselves some self-compassion.

SELF-KINDNESS

Allow your grief, in all its manifestations, to exist without feeling pressure to grieve in a certain way. Forgive yourself if you don't have the same energy as before. Listen to your body and, if you feel exhausted, let yourself sleep as much as you need to without feeling guilty. Cut yourself some much-needed slack where you can. If you feel foggy and disconnected, remind yourself that you're grieving and that everything you're experiencing is because your mind and body are functioning in survival mode.

COMMON HUMANITY

The exhaustion, the brain fog, the anxiety – *everything* you're feeling is a normal response to grief. On those days when it feels all too difficult and like you're living on a completely different planet from the rest of the world, remind yourself that you are not alone. The grief you're feeling is a normal human experience that is ultimately shared by everybody.

MINDFULNESS

Acknowledge how you're feeling. Bring awareness to whatever physical symptoms you're experiencing and accept that this is your reality in this present moment. It's awful, it's painful, and sometimes really frightening, but try to remember that these feelings are temporary.

Whatever you do, know that it's okay if you don't have the energy to go, go, go. It's okay if all you did today was survive. You're doing your best under extremely difficult circumstances.

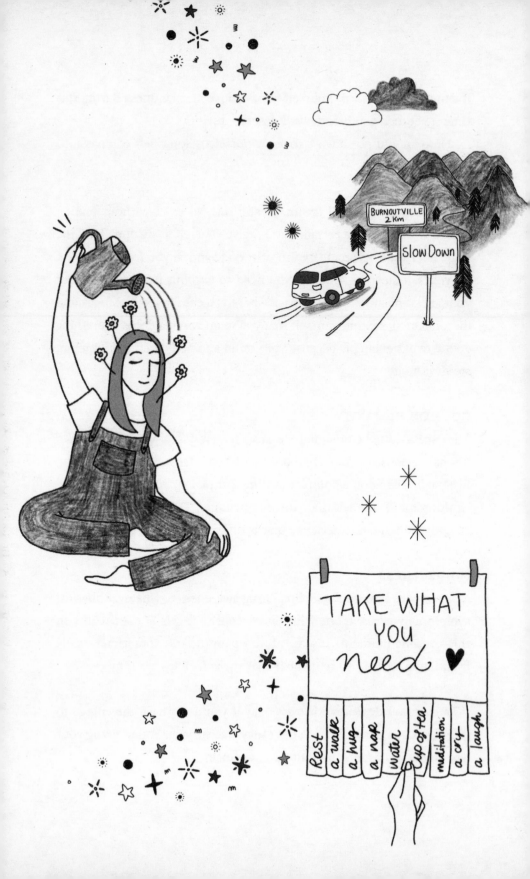

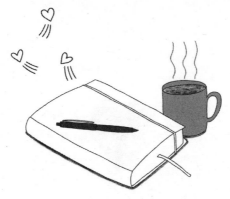

4.
SELF-CARE
FOR
GRIEVERS

How small changes can help you face each day

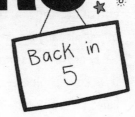

Back in 5

GRIEF IS ALL-CONSUMING AND OVERWHELMING.

As well as coping with the unrelenting emotional and physical impacts of grief, there are often loads of added pressures to contend with, such as returning to work, raising children, studying and running a household. If you are in the early stages of your loss, you may be having to deal with even more added stress – funeral planning, managing the estate or sorting out finances. It's a lot.

After someone dies, self-care can end up at the bottom of your priority list. Because let's face it, the last thing you feel like doing is looking after yourself when your whole world has imploded. Even meeting your most basic needs – things like remembering to drink water – can feel like an impossible task.

Self-care in grief isn't about face masks and massages. It's about survival. It's important to know how to replenish your reserves so that you can keep going. If you've been caring for someone who is at the end of life and you're coping with anticipatory grief, then your reserves might already be empty.

Learning what type of care to give yourself, and being realistic about it, is key. Implementing small changes in your day-to-day life after loss can play a fundamental role in how you cope.

Sal

As the sole executor of Mum's estate, it was on me to sort out everything, on top of coping with the shock of her death and my grief. It was incredibly confronting – no-one tells you that the amount of admin involved after someone dies is huge, and how it can add intense stress to the grieving process. There I was, not only trying to deal with my heartbreak, but also having to sort out Mum's estate, cancel her bills, bank accounts and subscriptions, plan her funeral, clear out her house, get estate agents round to value it . . . the list goes on. All of this was on top of supporting my autistic brother, my mum's partner and friends, and my aunts, uncles and cousins, who were all reeling from the shock of her death. Needless to say, I was totally overwhelmed, and I felt like I didn't have time to grieve properly. When I arrived back home in Australia, the admin involved in the estate continued to flow for a year after Mum's death. I had to sell her house from overseas and then the pandemic hit, which made things more challenging and distressing.

A 'doer' by nature, I project-managed my mum's estate like a pro – but it came at the expense of my wellbeing. I was stressed to the max, but I couldn't stop myself from trying to get it all done, going at full-speed even though I was an emotional mess and exhausted. This came to a head when I had a meltdown – life had become a never-ending to-do list. I was putting too much pressure on myself, not understanding that, in my grief, I wasn't able to whizz through tasks at the same speed as before. I was not okay, and what I needed was to allow more space to rest and give myself time to process what had happened.

I decided that I'd commit to 20 minutes of quiet 'me' time each evening to reflect and decompress, by journalling, reading, or connecting with my mum by looking at photos. This small shift genuinely made a difference to how I was then able to cope with the demands of daily life.

BURNOUT IN GRIEF

In some cases, grief can lead us beyond feeling overwhelmed to burnout. Burnout is defined by the American Psychological Association as 'physical, emotional, or mental exhaustion accompanied by decreased motivation, lowered performance and negative attitudes towards yourself, and others'. It occurs when stress and tension that are caused by a continued high performance level take their toll. It's not always easy to spot when you're close to burning out because, frankly, grief is already exhausting.

If you're worried you're speeding towards burnoutville, here are some signs to look for.

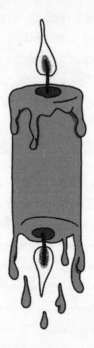

FEELING EXHAUSTED EMOTIONALLY, PHYSICALLY AND MENTALLY, TO THE POINT WHERE PERFORMING BASIC TASKS IS DIFFICULT

GETTING EASILY IRRITATED

LOSING DRIVE OR MOTIVATION

BECOMING INCREASINGLY CYNICAL

EXPERIENCING CONFLICT WITH FAMILY, FRIENDS OR COLLEAGUES

LACKING ANY EMPATHY OR EMOTION

UNABLE TO FOCUS OR CONCENTRATE

TACKLING GRIEF OVERWHELM

We talked about cognitive fatigue in Chapter 3, and how there are days when it can be hard to even think straight. The stress of trying to survive grief is physically exhausting – it takes insurmountable amounts of energy to process loss. When a hundred things are fighting for your mental attention and you're trying to cope with both grief and daily life, it can show up in different ways, including being snappy, tearful or angry, or lacking empathy for others. If you're feeling this way, then allowing yourself to rest and recharge – or simply grieve – is crucial.

It's time to get real about what's important, and what's not, as well as in which areas you might be able to ask for support. If you are feeling overwhelmed, or like you are heading towards burnout, here are some ideas on how to create more space for yourself.

Is it *really* that important?

Sometimes there's loads of admin that needs to be done after a death, and it's all important. When it comes to the day-to-day stressors, a good place to start is by brain-dumping everything that's on your to-do list, along with all the things that are overwhelming you. It's okay if it's pages long – you don't have to make a massive dent in the list, just get it all out as a starting point.

Once you have it all down, ask yourself what three things must get done today. The goal is to assess your to-do list based on priorities and figure out what you're unnecessarily piling your plate with. Does it *really* need to happen, or can you drop the ball on this one? Everything can feel important, but not everything is necessary right now. Grab a marker and highlight the three things that need to happen today, setting aside whatever can wait. This can help alleviate some of the pressure and might free up a bit of space in your day for self-care.

Who can help?

After a loss, people often say, 'Let me know how I can help!' Although you might not want to be a burden, right now you probably need all the help you can get, so seize the opportunity. If you have people you can rely on and trust, delegate things on your to-do list that will free up time to focus on yourself. People can feel helpless in the face of someone's grief, so being able to take on practical tasks, big or small, is a way of showing their care for you.

Some tasks that you could ask for help with are:

- **Communication** – is there someone who can act as a point person, to share important details with others, such as funeral arrangements?
- **Settling the estate** – are there some ways that others might be able to help, such as making phone calls, posting letters, or researching any information you need?
- **Cleaning** – is there a friend or family member who might be able to help you clean the house, or sort laundry?
- **Grocery shopping** – could someone do this for you, if you give them a list?
- **Childcare** – is there anyone who might be able to babysit for a few hours so that you can rest? Or someone who could do the school drop-off and pick-up for a week?
- **Dog walking** – do you have a friend who has a dog and could walk your dog, too?

What are two things that you need to do that you could ask for help with? Who can you ask?

Focus on what you can control

After a loss, it can feel like you don't have much control over your circumstances, and that can be incredibly stressful. When things get too much, it can be helpful to think about what you *can* control. Honestly, on really awful days, reminding yourself that there *are* things within your power can make a difference.

Here are some things that you can control:

- your words and actions
- the way you treat yourself and others
- your choices
- your response to other people's actions
- how you let other people affect you
- when (and if) you forgive others
- where you direct your time and energy
- boundaries you set with others.

What our community said about . . .

GRIEF OVERWHELM

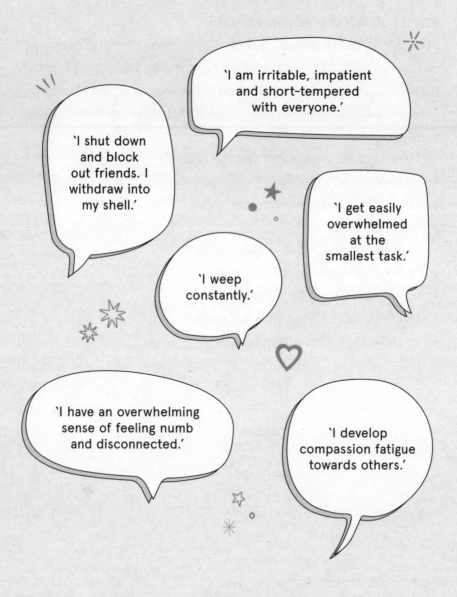

'I am irritable, impatient and short-tempered with everyone.'

'I shut down and block out friends. I withdraw into my shell.'

'I get easily overwhelmed at the smallest task.'

'I weep constantly.'

'I have an overwhelming sense of feeling numb and disconnected.'

'I develop compassion fatigue towards others.'

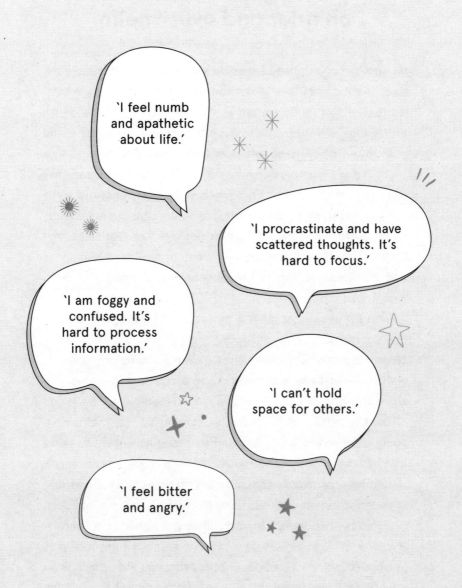

Psychologist Tamara's view on grief and overwhelm

My number one tip is to set aside a small window of time each day for your grief, and allow yourself to be lost in its waves. It is easier to function when you've acknowledged the depth of the loss. Often, trying to suppress grief means that it will pop up out of the blue and overwhelm you.

There are many free and accessible options for you that can support you in your grief journey. Several beneficial tools include spending time in nature, self-acceptance, exercising, avoiding drugs and alcohol, getting regular sleep, eating healthy foods, relaxation techniques (e.g. deep breathing, mindfulness and positive thinking), and seeking help and connection from your social circle.

Mindfulness is achieved by focusing awareness on the present moment, while accepting feelings, thoughts and bodily sensations non-judgementally. One easy way to practise this is with colouring in, which asks us to focus on how we choose and apply colour to a design. Similar to meditation, we let go of any thoughts about tomorrow or yesterday, or what we are going to do when we finish, and as thoughts enter the mind they are curiously watched without overly engaging with them.

Another technique is to cultivate self-acceptance. Be as kind to yourself as you are to others, by working on developing an inner voice that speaks to yourself as you would to a friend – less of a critic and more of a 'cheerleader'. See any mistakes as opportunities to learn, acknowledging you are human – we are not designed to get things 'right' all the time. Acknowledge and record the things you do well, however small.

BOUNDARIES

A big part of tackling overwhelm in grief (and possibly helping to prevent burnout) is setting boundaries. They can be a game changer because they help you to say no to things, people or situations for which you don't have the time or energy.

Before our losses, neither of us knew much about boundaries and would overstretch ourselves, often to our own detriment. Boundaries are not about saying no to everything or being harsh; they are healthy ways to create space for yourself. You might be on the receiving end of unsolicited advice, people might pry or ask uncomfortable questions, or you might be navigating unhealthy relationships with others. All of these can be helped by being honest, upfront and setting boundaries.

In her excellent book *Set Boundaries, Find Peace: A guide to reclaiming yourself*, therapist Nedra Glover Tawwab describes boundaries as the expectations and needs that help you feel safe and comfortable in your relationships, which in turn aid you in staying mentally and emotionally well. Why do we need boundaries in grief? If we don't set boundaries, we might neglect our self-care, resent others for asking for our help, avoid social interactions and generally feel overwhelmed and burnt out.

It's not always easy to set a boundary. It's natural to worry about how someone will respond, or whether it's the right thing to do. While it might feel uncomfortable at first, learning how to identify and create a boundary can make a big difference in tackling feelings of overwhelm. There's no definitive list of what you can set griefy boundaries around, but a good place to start is by thinking about areas at home, work or in your community where you might have felt stress or tension.

Boundaries in grief can look like:

- saying 'no' to a plan if you don't feel up to it
- not always being available if you need space

- limiting time with people who don't make you feel good
- dividing the workload at home
- letting people know when you don't want to talk about your loss
- letting people know when you don't want physical contact, such as hugs
- saying no to working overtime if you're feeling exhausted.

When we spoke to body-positivity advocate, author and manifestation coach Allira Potter, she shared how important setting boundaries has been to help her through the loss of her mum. She made a good point that, in the age of social media, we're used to instant gratification, and this extends to how boundary-less we've become. We often react straight away to questions or invitations from others, which means we say yes to things that we don't actually want to do, or that drain us. She suggests that next time someone asks you to do something, or go somewhere, pause to think about whether you want to do it. Do you have the capacity to do it right now? Will it make you feel good, or more stressed? If it's not a hard 'yes', she suggests it should be a firm, 'no, thanks'.

If you are keen to learn more about boundaries, we highly recommend Nedra's book and her Instagram account @nedratawwab, both of which have loads of great tips on setting healthy boundaries. Allira also has some great content about setting boundaries and you can find her on Instagram at @allira.potter.

What areas in your life do you feel are busting your boundaries? Where could you create a bit of space? Think about what drains you and what energises you.

Here are some examples of ways you could respectfully set a boundary

When you're given unsolicited advice . . . → 'I'm not seeking any advice right now. It would mean so much to me if you could listen without trying to offer a solution.'

When you don't feel like talking about your loss . . . → 'It's too hard for me to talk about it right now, but I appreciate you asking.'

When you're asking for support . . . → 'I'm struggling at the moment with _____. I need you to _____.' (e.g. 'take charge of making dinner this week').

When you're asked to do something you don't want to do . . . → 'I'll need to sleep on that and come back to you in the morning.'

When you want to say 'no' to an invitation . . . → 'Thanks for thinking of me. I've got a lot on my plate right now, so I'm going to have to say "no" this time.'

When people make assumptions about how you're coping . . . → 'I need you to understand that I am dealing with this at my own pace.'

What our community said about . . .

BOUNDARIES

'I had to let go of unnecessary obligations outside of my own home after my son died. I just needed to focus on taking care of myself. Because I knew if I didn't, I wouldn't be able to care for my family.'

'I ignored my own needs in my grief for the first nine months. I recently decided I had to reassess and set boundaries.'

'Experiencing multiple traumatic losses, many people wanted me to "get over" it. I have had to set boundaries between myself and these people and put my mental health first. It can be lonely, but it is so, so important.'

'I held so much space for other people's grief, but I felt like no-one held space for me. So, I had to set some boundaries to protect my energy.'

'I had to set boundaries with my best friend. She was dumping all her problems on me and it was too much for me to handle in my grief.'

Boundary busters

OVERLOADING YOUR
SCHEDULE

SPENDING TIME WITH
NEGATIVE PEOPLE

SCROLLING ON
SOCIAL MEDIA

ANSWERING
UNCOMFORTABLE
QUESTIONS

NEGATIVE SELF-TALK

PEOPLE-PLEASING
AND SAYING 'YES'

STAYING UP LATE

GOING TO SOCIAL
EVENTS WHEN
YOU'RE TIRED

AVOIDING YOUR
EMOTIONS

TAKING ON TOO
MANY TASKS

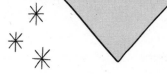

Boundary boosters

GIVING
YOURSELF
TIME TO REST

BEING WITH PEOPLE
WHO SUPPORT YOU

LIMITING SOCIAL
MEDIA USE

CHOOSING WHAT
QUESTIONS YOU
ANSWER

TALKING NICELY
TO YOURSELF

PUTTING YOUR
NEEDS FIRST

MAKING SLEEP
NON-NEGOTIABLE

BEING REALISTIC
ABOUT WHAT YOU
CAN DO

TRYING MEDITATION
AND JOURNALLING

ASKING FOR HELP

Im

Juggling grief and motherhood has been challenging. After Mum died, I was so focused on trying to look after my baby that my needs were coming last. I felt overwhelmed, exhausted, irritable and completely burnt out. I felt like I wasn't a 'good enough' mum because I didn't have a lot of patience. Some days the house was a mess, and the mental capacity to remember things like dress-up days at day care was non-existent. Cue mum guilt.

I wasn't giving myself enough grace. Being a first-time mum while grieving your own mum is hard work. My mum was my go-to for all things motherhood. When I hadn't slept all night and my cup was empty, she was the one who would fill it up with the reassurance and guidance that I desperately needed. Even the simple text messages she would send me, telling me how hard being a mum is and what an amazing job I was doing, lifted my self-doubt. I've gone to pick up the phone many times to ask her silly little questions about babies that I knew she'd have the answer to, and realising I couldn't ask her really hurt. Losing your mother can be a pivotal, life-changing moment for women. When you are trying to raise children of your own in the midst of grief, you can be met with many painful realisations.

No matter who you are grieving, raising children after a loss is tough. All we can do is show up each day and give it our best. If you haven't done the washing in a week, it's okay. If all you have the energy to make for dinner is baked beans on toast, that's okay, too. Prioritising yourself sometimes is vital, so try to set aside as little as 30 minutes a day to do something that fills your cup. For me, a long, steaming hot bath does the trick. It's important to remember that there is no such thing as the perfect parent. If your life feels overshadowed by grief right now and your children are fed, loved and cared for, you're doing a good job.

CREATING AN 'ENERGY BUDGET'

We only have so much energy in a day and, when we are grieving, it can feel like a lot of it is spent processing emotions and other daily stressors. Protecting your energy is part of setting boundaries, and that starts with becoming more mindful about where you're spending it. The comedian Whitney Cummings calls it spending 'energy dollars', which is a great way to think about it.

Let's say you start the day with 100 coins in your energy budget. How are you going to spend them? For example, big things like sorting out admin, planning the funeral, sorting the estate, or spending time with a family member might result in spending 50 coins. You've got 50 coins left – where do they go? Checking social media might take up three coins, texting back and forth might take five, emailing might take ten and cooking dinner might take 20. Think about where your energy is being spent, and how you can budget it better. How often are you spending time with people who deplete you? Are you unconsciously doing things that are blowing through your budget, such as checking your phone all the time?

A good tip is to give yourself some buffer in your budget by thinking of tasks you can do in bulk. For example, if you're working, you could pick out your outfits on a Sunday evening for the week ahead, so you'll save energy coins deciding what to wear each day. Instead of cooking from scratch every day, you might bulk-cook some meals to last a few days. Rather than picking up your phone every time you get a notification, why not turn off the notifications and only check your phone a few times a day?

SOMETIMES THE MOST IMPORTANT THING YOU CAN DO IS

unplug

AND

slow down.

SELF-CARE IN GRIEF: WHY DO WE NEED IT?

The term 'self-care' might conjure up thoughts of self-indulgence, extravagance and unnecessary expense (all things we don't give two shits about when we are feeling so much pain). But actually, it's about topping yourself up with much-needed fuel. It's *far* more than just a cocktail, pamper session or hot bath (although they are nice things to have as part of your life, too). At its core, as the poet Audre Lorde wrote back in 1988, self-care is an act of self-preservation. It's about finding simple ways to help you survive the chaos that you find yourself in.

When you're feeling less than average, you might not have one ounce of energy or even the headspace to think about anything other than your loss. Even if you try to do things for yourself, it might feel too hard. We've been there – the stressed-out, trying-to-be-Zen-but-irritable-as-hell meditation sessions. Your needs take a back seat while you simply try to make sense of everything.

Caring for yourself starts with cultivating the habit of checking in with what's happening for you and then responding in the most loving way possible. It's a skill, but it doesn't need to be complicated or hard to master. Resting when you want to do that extra task but feel depleted, calling a friend and letting off some steam, asking for help, saying no to social activities that drain you and limiting screen time are all acts of caring for *you*.

It's not about adding more to your plate or giving up the things that give you a feeling of escapism, like Netflix marathons or enjoying a glass of wine with friends. It's figuring out what simple things you need to do to support yourself, in an achievable way. We're not advocating for an expensive new gym membership or day spa session, or doing something that is going to take time, money, energy or effort. Instead, it's all about using what little bandwidth you have to find small ways to care for yourself and make your situation a little more sustainable.

It took us both a good while to come to grips with how to properly nourish ourselves to better cope with our loss. It's something we are still working on, but mastering the art of authentic self-care has been important for us in our grief. When you know what you need to do to look after yourself, it can be transformative.

For Sal, self-care means:
- reading a chapter of a book
- going for a walk outside
- switching her phone to 'do not disturb' in the evenings.

For Im, self-care means:
- limiting alcohol
- doing 15 minutes of boxing or going for a run
- listening to a calming meditation to fall asleep.

By paying attention to your needs, you are building the ability to listen to yourself, which is a great act of kindness to you, and a small but necessary foundation for healing when you are grieving. It's really about figuring out a simple framework that you can include in your day-to-day routine to help you manage stress better and increase your resilience and strength.

You don't have to feel like you're floating on a cloud or have mastered inner peace (although both would be great!). Being there for yourself in gentle and compassionate ways can create coping mechanisms that support you in feeling calm, and add more balance. So, if you feel like you don't have time to prioritise yourself, think again. This is *essential* to your healing.

Kelley's experience with self-care

'After my mom died, sorting out the "business" of death fell on my shoulders. In the first month, I was the busiest I have ever been – my adrenaline-driven state felt like an out-of-body experience. Yet, as I tried to get it all done in a state of shock, I went from maximum productivity to full-body burnout, which left me incapable of even minor tasks. It took more than six months for me to feel capable of returning to work after hitting rock bottom, and even then it was in a limited capacity. It's completely changed how I operate – I've still yet to reach my former efficiency level without finding myself completely exhausted.'

What helped

'Advocating for my self-care has been so important, as well as recognising that the little energy I have is very precious. I created a budget for my energy and I stick to it religiously – I've had to evaluate all my relationships and determine how much attention I can afford to expend on those around me. For me, burnout led to the ultimate crash course in setting boundaries and sticking to them.'

CARING FOR YOURSELF WHEN YOU'RE A CARER

If you're responsible for caring for others, then carving out chunks of time for yourself isn't realistic. You might not have periods of time alone where you can focus on loss, or grieve, and instead must just 'get on with it'.

When we spoke to Huntington's Disease advocate Kelly Terranova about her experience of caring for her mum, she explained the importance of being realistic about the toll that caring for someone takes on you. For Kelly, if she does a long care shift for her mum, she knows she won't be able to perform the next day. So, rather than trying to move at the same pace, she accepts that it won't all get done and puts a plan in place. Staying organised can help you feel in control – for example, having a planner, or keeping a schedule of your routine.

Instead of trying to find the magic cure for the pain of her mum dying and the stress of seeing her upset, Kelly also chooses to accept that the pain isn't going away. Instead, she looks for tiny moments of self-care that help keep her afloat. That might be making her mum her favourite soup, or buying her favourite coffee after a long care shift.

 Let others in on the act. Tell your partner, family, friends or colleagues your intention to incorporate more self-care into your life. Let them know it's okay to give you some extra encouragement to do the small things that make you feel good, especially on tough days.

CREATING SELF-CARE 'MICRO-RITUALS'

We all have those griefy days when everything feels too much. When they hit, it's important to have self-care 'tools' that boost your wellbeing, but require minimal effort. When life is busy, coping strategies need to be realistic. A good way to think about incorporating some self-care into your day is to create very small 'micro-rituals' that you can do for yourself when you have little scraps of time to spare. It's not about trying to overstretch yourself – it might be a few minutes after you wake up, or five minutes before you go to bed. A little bit of time each day can make a positive difference. Some things might work well on some days and not on others, so it's good to identify a few.

Here are some micro-rituals you could try.

- Make a cup of your favourite tea. Sit and drink it without any distractions.
- Drink a glass of lemon water as soon as you wake up, to start your day hydrated.
- On a nice day, go and sit with your face in the sun for a few minutes.
- Take time to read a few pages of a novel (ideally something non-griefy!).
- Use your favourite moisturiser to give yourself a hand massage.
- Do some gentle yoga stretches for a few minutes.
- Eat a square of your favourite chocolate – really relish it.
- Take a few minutes to play with your pet.
- Create a mini bedtime facial routine, and make it feel like you're in a spa.
- Inhale a smell that uplifts you. Try lavender, peppermint or sage.
- Before you go to sleep, take a few minutes to write down one thing that you appreciate.

What our community said about . . .

THEIR FAVOURITE WAYS TO PRACTISE SELF-CARE

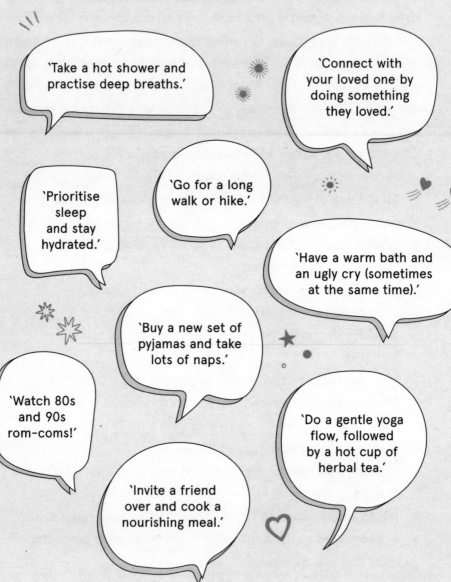

'Take a hot shower and practise deep breaths.'

'Connect with your loved one by doing something they loved.'

'Prioritise sleep and stay hydrated.'

'Go for a long walk or hike.'

'Have a warm bath and an ugly cry (sometimes at the same time).'

'Buy a new set of pyjamas and take lots of naps.'

'Watch 80s and 90s rom-coms!'

'Do a gentle yoga flow, followed by a hot cup of herbal tea.'

'Invite a friend over and cook a nourishing meal.'

It's time to create your self-care plan. Using the ideas from this chapter, think about what self-care rituals you'd like to incorporate. In your journal, create four columns: Physical, Emotional, Spiritual and Social. List the things you think will help you in each area.

Some useful questions to ask yourself include:
* *what makes me feel relaxed?*
* *what makes me feel connected?*
* *what makes me feel supported?*
* *is there anything that has worked for me in the past?*
* *how much time do I have available to give myself?*

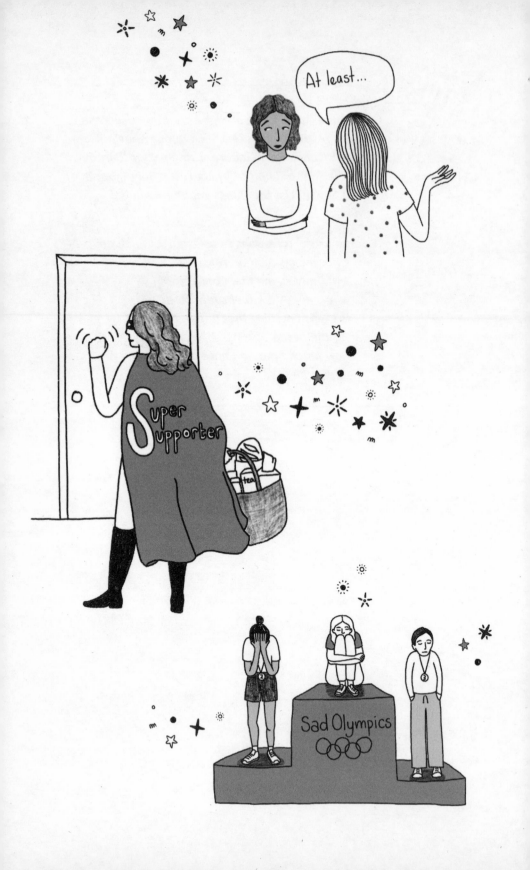

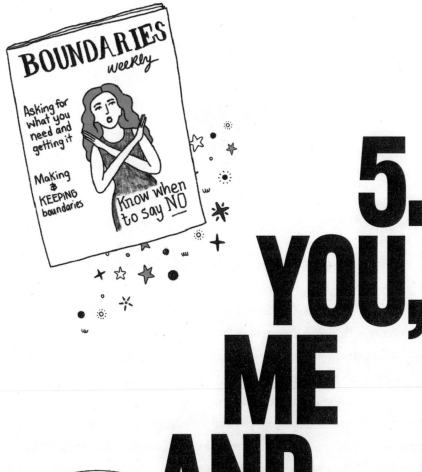

5.
YOU, ME AND GRIEF

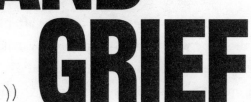

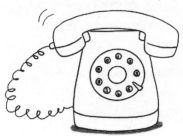

A deep dive into how grief impacts relationships

LOSS CAN SHINE A SPOTLIGHT ON THE RELATIONSHIPS IN YOUR LIFE.

Loss illuminates people's best and worst traits and it can cause ruptures and rifts, challenging all types of bonds (no matter how strong they are). As if grieving isn't enough on its own, maintaining relationships after a loss can be exhausting.

When grief strikes, it can shake up your support system. At a time when you sure as hell need all the support you can get, not everyone is prepared to meet you in your pain. Some people show up, while others check out. If the ones who checked out are the very same people you thought would help keep you afloat, that can come as a major shock.

We all cope differently in times of crisis, and this can be a big factor when it comes to relationship changes after loss. No two people grieve in the same way – some find comfort in talking about the person who died, others avoid mentioning them at all. You may even end up in a game of 'who's pain is the worst?' (because 'competitive grief' is absolutely a thing). It's almost impossible for us to nail down all the different scenarios. However, when people around you aren't providing a safe and supportive space to express your grief, or they are dishing out unhelpful platitudes because they don't know what else to say, it can make you feel super lonely and compound your sense of loss.

Even though people can be rubbish when it comes to grief support, with a little bit of patience and understanding, it is possible to rebuild bridges that may have been burnt along the way. Equally, grief can make us re-evaluate the kinds of relationships we want in our lives, and sometimes, re-inventing your support circle may be the best thing for you. Whatever your circumstances, making sure you stay true to yourself and your needs is top priority.

WHEN YOUR SUPPORT TEAM CHANGES

One of the biggest surprises for grievers is that it's not always the people who you *think* will be there who show up for you after a loss. The days and weeks after a death can be flooded with commiserations, but after the funeral, support can drop off. Your closest allies might have no clue what to say. The phone calls and texts dry up, and you find yourself looking at your once-on-speed-dial phone contacts and wondering where they are.

There's nothing like death to render people silent. Perhaps because it's so confronting, and permanent, even the best communicators can end up dumbstruck. A tweet by the author and grief expert Megan Devine said that 'grief changes your address book', and she's spot on. Grief rearranges some relationships – people can, and do, drop away. The people who you thought would be the first to offer a listening ear or sit with you in the front row at the funeral might be distant. They might tiptoe around the topic awkwardly, flake on plans, say insensitive stuff or make your loss all about them. A lot of people also don't know how to, or if they even should, bring up your loss. They might not mention your person, change the subject, or act miffed that you're still grieving months or years on. In some cases, they disappear entirely, without explanation.

All of this can be hard to swallow. Friends dropping away and family members falling silent is a common grief experience, and it really hurts. If they're uncomfortable with grief, or can't grasp the enormity of your loss, it might feel like an extra effort for them to maintain the connection. They might not make space for you to talk about your loss, and all of this can be baffling.

On the other end of the spectrum, some people are brilliant and fly in like superheroes. They always check-in and seem to know exactly what you need at any moment. It's not always the people you've known the longest, either. Casual acquaintances can become your best supporters. People from the past can resurface and those relationships might be renewed.

As human beings, we are wired to connect with others, and social support is important when coping with loss. If your connections aren't meeting your needs and you don't feel like you are understood in your grief, it's a lonely place to be. What's more, the secondary losses of changing relationships can feel like grief layered on top of grief, which is no fun for anyone. When you expect your closest confidants to be there for you, you may experience feelings of anger, shame and disappointment if they don't have your back.

When other people let you down when you need them the most, it can lead you to reassess those relationships. The energy and time you have to invest in them might shrink, or some things that you accepted from them in the past just don't cut the mustard anymore. It's okay if the relationship is beyond repair and you don't want to give people second (or third) chances. If someone is harmful, emotionally draining or manipulative, it may be time to cut ties entirely.

One thing that has helped us is to remember that people can only meet you and your pain as deeply as they've met themselves. Not everyone is prepared to handle your grief or has the capacity to give you the support you deserve. Grief is often invisible to others – people are so caught up in their own lives that they might not see how deep the pain of grief runs, or not realise that grief isn't a three-week stint that goes away after the funeral. It's not an excuse for others, but it can help keep you sane when you feel let down.

After our mums died, we both found that because few of our peers had experienced grief in their thirties, they didn't quite understand the extent of what we were going through. They were supportive in ways, but through no fault of their own, not all of them knew what to do or say. Even with the best intentions, it's often not until you've experienced grief that you really 'get it'. Also, whether they've gone through a loss or not, some people just aren't skilled in providing emotional support or don't have the bandwidth due to personal reasons. If people have been there for you but maybe not to the extent you'd hoped, sometimes it's helpful to let them off the hook with a bit of forgiveness or lower your expectations – because we're all learning about grief as we go.

GRIEF TIP

Although people might not know how to support you, it doesn't necessarily mean that they don't want to. It can help to actively let others know what you need. If that's a listening ear, tell them that you don't need any advice right now, you just want someone to share your thoughts with. If you are feeling overwhelmed and need some practical help, ask them if they have any spare time to help you with some tasks. You may not feel like you have the energy to have these types of conversations face to face, so communicating your needs via text is totally acceptable.

What our community said about . . .

COPING WITH A LACK OF SUPPORT

'Protect your energy. Insensitive interactions are draining!'

'Focus on showing gratitude for the ones who are there for you. Forget the rest.'

'Strengthen the good existing relationships, even if it's only one or two.'

'Put you and your needs first. If someone is making things worse, they aren't worth your time.'

'Learn to be okay with letting go of relationships that aren't genuine, and try not to be angry about it.'

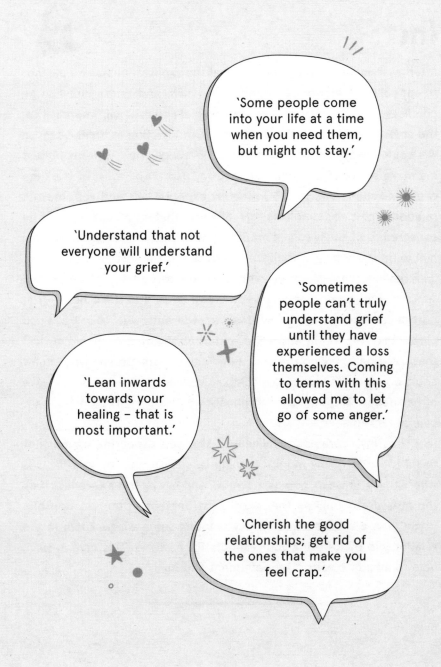

Im

After my mum died, I put a lot of unrealistic expectations on my partner to support me emotionally (and financially), and that caused some conflict within our relationship. He is logical and rational, whereas I am the emotional one, and the dynamic caused friction at times because we would always be on two different levels of grief. Therapy helped me make sense of the situation, and my psychotherapist at the time explained that I needed to lower my expectations and reframe the relationship. It's as simple as that. She said that my partner cannot be expected to fill every role in my life, and that hit home. I was expecting him to be everything, and that's unrealistic in any sort of relationship.

I realised that Mum was the person I turned to for emotional support. Whenever anything went wrong in my life, she'd be my first port of call, and she somehow always knew exactly what to say. She had played that role for my entire life, and when she died, I completely lost that. I couldn't pick up the phone and call the one person who I knew could comfort me in the ways that I so very much needed in the wake of her death. And that unconditional love of a parent, unfortunately, cannot be replaced.

I took my therapist's advice and stopped expecting my partner to fill the role of my mum. Learning to self-soothe my grief (this is where the 'grief sesh' comes in handy), and having this awareness took the pressure off my partner and has strengthened our relationship. If you're in a similar situation, try creating some wiggle room in the relationship by lowering your expectations a little. This can, in turn, help to minimise your disappointment and hurt.

Sandra's experience with a lack of support

'My dad was diagnosed with lymphoma in September 2005, after a year of being sick. Five months later, he was transferred to a hospice and died within three days. I'd always been "Daddy's little girl", and my siblings teased me mercilessly for it growing up. After he died, I was unprepared for the recognition that I had no connection with my mum. Suddenly it was clear that Dad was my safety net – as long as he was around, I always knew I had a home and felt loved.

'My mum has struggled with mental illness and she spent a month institutionalised when I was one. This had a significant impact on my relationship with her. My dad was dependable, reliable, safe and my world, but the extent of this only became truly apparent to me after he died.

'Initially, following Dad's death, I tried to force a connection with Mum, but that did not work – it only amplified my grief and I felt as if I was being disloyal to my dad. We also had some very tense and awkward conversations. I was struggling with my grief, and trying to get support from my mum made me feel worse.'

What helped

'With the help of therapy, I've learned to stop trying to force a connection. I accept that our relationship has limitations. We don't have a strong bond and I can't rely on my mum for support, but that's okay – I have other support systems. I miss my dad, but I'll treasure our connection until the day I die.'

PLATITUDE-FREE ZONE

Another big reason for feeling less-than supported in your relationships is receiving unhelpful platitudes. You know – the meaningless clichés, offhand comments and ill-fitting statements that are often dished out automatically. They often include unsolicited advice about what you should or shouldn't do. People might feel like they need to share their experience with loss; even if they have the best intentions, it can feel like your loss is being compared to theirs, or not acknowledged at all. You don't want to have to pretend you are doing okay, to be told 'you'll be all right', or 'stay strong'. You probably don't want to give a polite smile and nod along to 'at least they're in a better place', either.

Part of what makes platitudes so difficult to hear is that they are often out of alignment with what you are feeling. Dismissive statements can feel minimising for a griever, as if the words are expected to instantly lessen your pain, when in reality all they do is take away the opportunity for you to be vulnerable. You grin and bear it so you don't make the situation uncomfortable for the other person, although, no doubt, you'd rather flip them the middle finger!

Grief is hard, but you don't need to be told how to make it better, you need support to get through it. You don't need platitudes right now (or ever) – you need to feel understood and to have space to just be.

A brilliant piece of advice when it comes to handling platitudes comes from our community member, Stacey. She suggests that, when hit by griefy platitudes, ask yourself: *Is this hurtful or helpful?* When a hurtful statement comes your way, you need to protect your energy by advocating for yourself. Set the record straight, in a polite but firm way – it's okay to let people know if their comments hurt. Maybe the next time that person comes into contact with someone else going through loss, they will have a better understanding of what *not* to say.

What our community said about . . .

THEIR EXPERIENCE WITH PLATITUDES

'I buried my little sister and my older brother this summer. Being told "God needed them more" pissed me off no end – as if their kids, who were just babies, didn't need them as well.'

'My dad died very unexpectedly three years ago at the young age of 62. People said all kinds of unhelpful things to my family. My dad was 62! It didn't feel like it was "his time to go". People also said, "He's in a better place." While I'm a Christian, I still wondered what was so wrong with being here with his family where he belongs?'

'Although always well-intended, I find "she is watching over you" really isolating because I simply don't believe that. I think it also disables me from talking bluntly about my grief. An open question like, "What do you think your mum would think?" would be much more helpful.'

'My brother died recently, and everyone has been saying he's in a better place or that it was God's plan. It makes me feel awful.'

'About ten weeks after losing my husband, someone in my family asked me if I had anything exciting to tell them. I just looked at her in disbelief.'

Here are some responses you could try next time a platitude comes your way

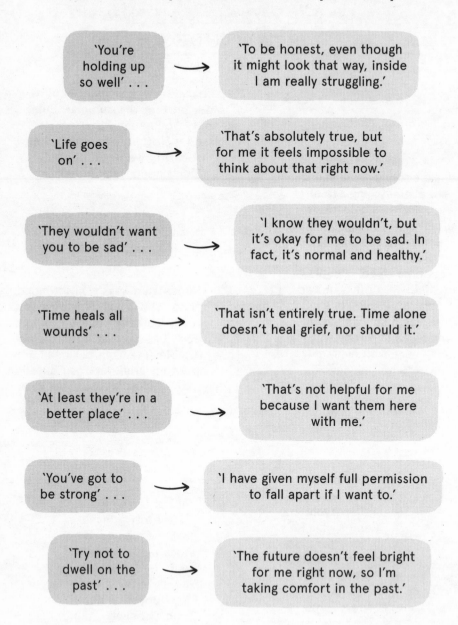

'You're holding up so well' . . . → 'To be honest, even though it might look that way, inside I am really struggling.'

'Life goes on' . . . → 'That's absolutely true, but for me it feels impossible to think about that right now.'

'They wouldn't want you to be sad' . . . → 'I know they wouldn't, but it's okay for me to be sad. In fact, it's normal and healthy.'

'Time heals all wounds' . . . → 'That isn't entirely true. Time alone doesn't heal grief, nor should it.'

'At least they're in a better place' . . . → 'That's not helpful for me because I want them here with me.'

'You've got to be strong' . . . → 'I have given myself full permission to fall apart if I want to.'

'Try not to dwell on the past' . . . → 'The future doesn't feel bright for me right now, so I'm taking comfort in the past.'

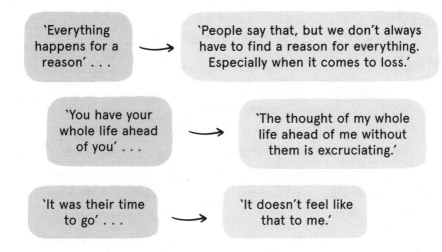

Grace's experience with platitudes

'I lost my partner, Ryan, to a rare form of soft-tissue cancer called synovial sarcoma when he was 28. Hearing platitudes is tough: "Oh, you are so young! You will find someone else for sure.", "At least you didn't have children/get married/own a house together. How difficult would all that paperwork be to sort out?" or "Ryan wouldn't want you to be sad. Get out there and live your life!"

'I understand that these comments are well-meaning and if said by loved ones they come from a place of love and support. But in the deepest, darkest depths of despair in grief, they are extremely unhelpful. Grief cannot be fixed, even with all the best intentions – I am hurting, and will continue to hurt from Ryan's loss until my time on this earth has come to an end.' →

What helped

◁

'A practical tip I have learned is, when these comments come your way, speak your truth. Don't be afraid to tell that person that their platitude, right now, is unhelpful. This could go along the lines of, "I appreciate you wanting to help me through this, but this is something that cannot be fixed and I need to experience my grief my way." The more you speak about your grief, the more you help others better understand how to be there for you.'

EVERYONE COPES DIFFERENTLY

Do you feel like you are grieving differently compared to everyone around you? Perhaps you've been caught up in disputes and differing opinions over money, funeral plans, wills and estates? If you're nodding, you are not alone. Disagreements are often inevitable when everyone is exhausted and emotions are running high.

A huge pain point in relationships after death is that we all express our grief differently, which can lead to misunderstandings. Loss can flip the script on how people normally behave and it can come as a big surprise when the people you're closest to react in a way you don't expect. Sometimes it can even feel like you're in a whole new relationship. If dynamics have shifted and your grief isn't being understood or recognised with compassion, you might not have the headspace or patience to cope.

There are so many layers that exist between two people that influence how grief is felt, and responded to. As challenging as it is when you don't see eye to eye with others, it's important to remember, as we explored in

Chapter 1, that there can be different grieving styles that influence how people express grief. A good piece of advice that author David Kessler shared with us that might help you to reframe how you approach the way others are grieving is to come from a place of compassion. You can't 'fix' the other person or change how they respond, but you can try to understand them. As much as you might question whether they are coping in the right way, as we have already mentioned, there's no *right* way to do any of this. According to David, 'There is no such thing as one person crying too much or one person crying too little – your crying or not crying is just right for you.'

Natalie's experience with a partner who coped differently

'Our beautiful baby boy passed away at just four days old. My partner and I were in shock. For the first few weeks, we comforted each other. But, as weeks went by, our different grieving styles turned us against each other. He was trying to be the "strong man" and didn't show much emotion. I was the opposite to him – a heartbroken, crying wreck.

'All my friends and family were around, sending me flowers, food, gifts, cards and messages. My partner hardly got any support from his family or friends, which was hard to watch. A few weeks later, he went back to work while I stayed home. I had visitors coming over asking what had happened and by the time he got home from work each day, I was a mess. He wanted me to have no visitors because it upset me to relive the trauma, but I needed people around. We would argue; —▷

◁ he was angry that I was so upset after having people here and he was sick of visitors.

'After a few more weeks of living through hell, I woke up one day feeling different. I thought, *What would my son think of me right now?* I had to change. I planned a trip to the beach to visit my two sisters and ended up staying there for two months. I realised that my partner and I needed space to breathe, miss each other and grieve differently in our own time.'

What helped

'My advice for couples grieving the loss of a child is to let each other breathe. Sometimes space helps, even if it's just for a few days. Remember that your partner can't fix everything – you need a whole network of family and friends to support you, not just one person who is broken, too.'

Communicating when you're coping differently

It's not always easy to state your needs when you're deep in grief. But, no matter your coping style, it's important to be able to express your thoughts and feelings safely.

One helpful tool when asking for what you need from others is the 'D-E-A-R M-A-N' exercise. It's a component of dialectical behavioural therapy (DBT), which is a form of cognitive behavioural therapy (CBT), that was developed by Dr Marsha Linehan to help people communicate their needs and resolve conflict in a way that maintains the relationship. What's great about it is that it can help you develop the skills to deal with highly emotional circumstances, such as conflict in grieving styles. It's a good idea to talk to the other person face to face if possible, as it can be easy to misinterpret what people are saying if you can't read their body language or see their facial expressions.

Here's how it works.

Describe the current situation, sticking only to the facts.

Express how the situation made you feel, as this will help the other person understand why the situation matters to you. Don't assume that they know how you feel!

Assert yourself by letting them know exactly what you want. Be specific and don't assume that they can read your mind!

Reinforce by focusing on what the positive effects will be from you getting what you want or need. Do it with a smile because that often helps.

Mindfulness means staying focused on the situation at hand. Keep focused on your goal and don't go off topic. You might feel like a broken record, but it's important to get your point across.

Appear confident. You may feel like a blubbering mess inside, but try to use a calm and clear tone, and make good eye contact. Own it!

Negotiate and remember that you are asking for something, not demanding it. Be open to offering solutions, or a compromise to solve the problem another way.

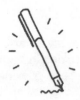

Think about a conversation that you could have using the 'D-E-A-R M-A-N' tool. What could you say? What would the desired outcome be?

What our community said about . . .

DIFFERENT COPING STYLES

'My husband and I grieve very differently, and it's been a real challenge.'

'My parents are not dealing with their grief well at all and it is straining our relationship.'

'My mum was the one who facilitated our internal family dynamics. It's like we have been thrown in with a bunch of strangers and are learning how to be around each other.'

'My girlfriend seems to be "fine" after our friend died, and it's strained our relationship.'

'My son and daughter are complete opposites in how they are coping with my husband's death, and it's caused a lot of friction.'

'It's always me making an effort for my dad and checking in on him, even though we are both grieving. He is depressed, but it's so exhausting to be the only one trying, as I am struggling, too.'

Psychologist Tamara's view on different coping styles

If you are grieving alongside family and friends, there will probably be times when how you cope with your grief clashes with how someone is coping with theirs. Most people describe feeling their needs constantly change, one moment to the next. The chance that you are both experiencing the same feeling, at the same time, is incredibly unlikely.

As hard as it may be, it's important for family members to be open and honest when talking with each other. Acknowledge aloud to them that you are grieving differently and tell them what you need from them. For example, tell them it's okay for them to talk to you about the person you've lost, and that if you get upset, then that's okay, too. You can say something like, 'I'd like to talk about it. Do you mind listening?' If you need something specific, let your loved ones know, such as, 'I don't want to be alone. Could you keep me company for a while?'

Try to remember that everyone copes differently and, rather than arguing over who is hurting the most, a better solution would be to accept that each person is hurting and coping in their own way. However, if you're feeling completely unsupported in your grief, often called disenfranchised grief, it may be time to take some space from your loved ones. Don't apologise for grieving, and don't let others dictate whether or not you have a right to 'feel' your emotions. Try to free yourself from expectations and permit yourself to grieve in your own way and in your own time. You can decide at a later date whether the relationships are healthy for you; right now, take your time and some space if you need.

THE GRIEF OLYMPICS

Competitive grief? Yep, it's absolutely a thing, and it can span all types of relationships. As humans, we all want our pain to be seen and acknowledged. But sometimes, there can be a sense of someone's grief being more valid, or more important, based on their relationship with the person who died. This can leave others feeling like they don't qualify for support, or that their feelings or experiences don't matter.

As Megan Devine wrote in her article 'The Hierarchy of Grief: Some people are at the periphery', 'some are at the epicentre of loss, and some are not'. She's right – some people will be more impacted by the loss, depending on how interconnected their lives were. Some people's daily lives might radically shift and change, whereas others might only be impacted slightly. Yet, she also says, like some sort of 'Grief Olympics', people can (and do) compete for whose pain is worse, which can have significant effects on relationships. You might feel like people around you are shouting, 'The depth of my grief wins, a gold medal for me!' Cue fallouts, relationships shifting and people feeling that their pain is minimised, or that they have to make excuses for their feelings.

When your grief feels like it's being compared with others', it can be tricky emotional terrain to navigate. People might give attention to one person who is experiencing loss, and ignore you entirely. Or, you might find that you're pushing your grief, or right to grieve, aside and it gets relegated to the bottom of the pile. Author Nora Zelevansky explained that after one of her oldest, most kindred friends died, there was a desperate desire from those in her friendship circle to have their relationship's legitimacy with him confirmed over others'. People might try to 'one-up' you on how they feel, how much the person meant to them, or their overall experience with grief. Grief isn't a competition, though. No-one is going to get the title of 'World's Greatest Griever' because it doesn't exist. Everyone, despite the level of relationship they had with the person who died, deserves to have their grief acknowledged.

Grief is entirely personal and there's no bar to meet to qualify because everyone will feel varying shades of pain. There's no value in determining who is grieving the most. Your grief is valid, their grief is valid and there's no point trying to compare losses.

Sibling grief

There is one type of relationship that can be especially impacted by grief hierarchies, and that's the loss of a sibling. Sibling grief is largely under-acknowledged, misunderstood, downplayed or even overshadowed by the grief of other family members. Even though siblings often share the strongest of bonds, they are often referred to as the 'forgotten mourners'. It's common for people to ask how the parents are, but not the siblings. Despite sharing life-long bonds, the grief of an adult sibling can feel overshadowed by the parents, partners or children of the person who died. It can feel like your loss doesn't matter. It does.

We have heard sibling loss described as being like an amputation. Not only do siblings lose a connection to their past and present, but also the future. A sibling is a part of you that was always there – a shared history, shared memories and even shared opinions on family dynamics. For many, losing a sibling is out of the natural order of things, and that makes this type of loss hard to comprehend.

The death of a sibling can change the entire family dynamic. It's common for the surviving brothers or sisters to feel like they have to hold it together and 'be strong' for the rest of the family. There can also be the added pressure of feeling like you have to look after your parents after a sibling dies, or hold your grief in around them. None of this is easy, and if you're coping with the loss of a sibling and needing some extra support, siblinggriefclub.com is a fantastic resource.

What our community said about...

COMPETITIVE GRIEF

'My husband died, and a close friend of ours always implies his grief is worse than mine – it's infuriating!'

'Dad told us it's worse for Mum as she carried my brother.'

'My mother-in-law acts as if her grief trumps mine when it comes to the loss of *my* child.'

'I can't talk to my mum about my dad dying – she just fobs me off as if her grief is worse.'

'When my brother died, I felt like I wasn't allowed to grieve as much as his wife and kids.'

'I have family members who think they should be considered the "sadder" ones.'

'My partner always implies that she feels her grief more than me, and that's tough as I am in deep pain, too.'

'My dad thinks his grief is the hardest since Mum died. My youngest sister thinks she needs Mum the most; I am the eldest and the assumption is that it's easier for the eldest, but it's not the case at all.'

'Since Dad died, my sister seems to think that, because I don't cry all the time, I am not as sad as she is.'

'There's a lot of point-scoring between my kids as to who has the most grief.'

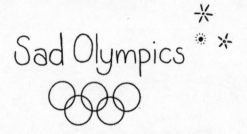

Sad Olympics

Kate's experience with competitive grief

'In January 2021, I lost my cousin, who was one of mine and my husband's best friends, in a car accident. Then, ten months later, I lost my big brother to an overdose. I like to make room for everyone and try to empathise with each family member who has lost their unique relationship with our loved ones. I've come to realise that even if you hold space for others, they might not do the same for you.

'When talking about my brother's death with some family members, I received hurtful comments such as, "Try being his [insert relationship]" or "You don't understand." I finally had the courage to say, "Help me understand" or "I can't try to be his [insert relationship] because I'm his sister." It felt like a competition.'

What helped

'If you're experiencing competitive grief, find your circle of friends who want to be supportive, even if they don't always know what to say. Those people are my safe haven, but they are not responsible for my grief and I make sure to make that clear.'

YOUR GRIEF

IS VALID.

We repeat:

YOUR GRIEF

IS VALID.

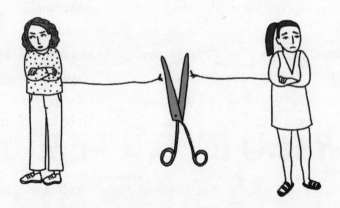

WHAT TO REMEMBER IF YOUR RELATIONSHIPS HAVE CHANGED

If you're experiencing changes in your relationships, it's not a reflection on you (or your grief). Here are some things to remember that can help when you're feeling relationship shifts and rifts.

- **It's okay if you don't want certain people in your life.**
  Grief changes our outlook, and priorities. If people haven't shown up for you, it's okay to implement boundaries or look for a new support network.
- **One person cannot be the sole provider of emotional support, so find an outside outlet.** If you're relying on someone for support but they don't understand how you're processing your grief, look to outside sources. Therapy and grief support groups can be a great place to start (more on that in Chapter 6).
- **Understand what you can control.** You can't control other people's reactions, but you can control your own. Just remembering this can help with your sanity when other people are pushing your buttons!

- **Try not to take 'negative' emotions personally.** Some people might be angry and express it loudly. Others might retreat inwards. The key is, don't take it personally, or react defensively against it. Grief means emotions are fully charged and can lead to hurtful things being said in the heat of the moment.
- **Accept your differences.** If someone seems to be expressing themselves emotionally in a different way, that's okay. Accept that that's them, and you do you.
- **Respond, don't react.** When dealing with difficult situations, it can be so easy to be reactive. But, for the sake of keeping the peace, overreacting may not be the best solution. If you can feel yourself getting worked up, take some deep breaths or go for a brisk walk around the block before you respond.
- **Practise forgiveness.** It's not always easy when people don't support us, or don't behave in the ways we'd hoped they would. Remember that not everyone is good at grief support – they simply may not have the skills to show up for you in this way, but it doesn't mean that they can't still play a role in your life.

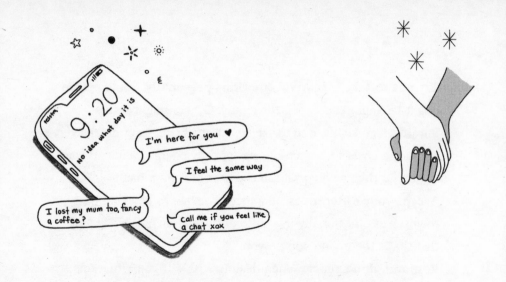

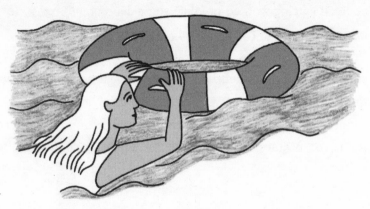

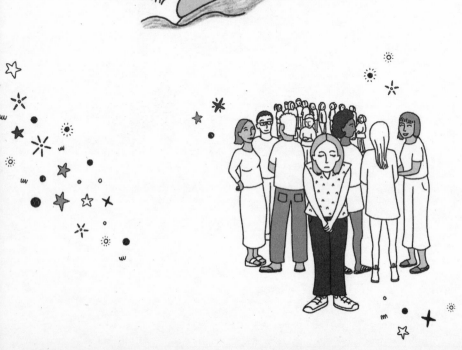

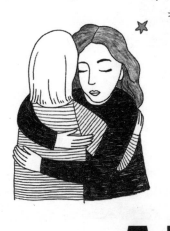

6.
YOU ARE NOT ALONE

Coping with loneliness after loss

GRIEF IS F*CKING LONELY.

When someone you love dies and your reality changes, it can feel like nobody understands the level of pain you are living with every day. Your world has come to a standstill, yet for everyone else it's business as usual. How can people around you be going about their day like everything is normal, when the worst possible thing has happened to you?

As we've explored, our relationships are central to coping with loss, yet they can also be a huge source of loneliness. We need each other to get through tough times, but so often in grief we are misunderstood – we're assumed to be broken or stuck if we're still feeling griefy a few months after the funeral (and sometimes even sooner). We're encouraged to put on a brave face and 'be strong'. And when you're always trying to fulfil that expectation and appear as if you're doing okay, your true state (aka the grieving you) isn't acknowledged. This can lead to feeling like you've got to cope with grief alone, when what you really need is support from people with a willingness to listen, along with permission to open up and let the pain of a loss unfurl in all its unpredictability.

Loneliness has played a huge part in our grief – without it, we wouldn't have met or written this book. We understand how isolating it feels, even with people around. As we've found, there's power in grief support and finding a community who 'get it'. Connecting to others who understand your pain can be key to living with loss. Grief is far too heavy to carry by yourself. And the good news is: you don't have to do it alone.

FEELING ADRIFT

After a loss it's common (and normal) to feel completely disconnected from your life and the people around you. The pain and gravity of grief is so huge that it can be hard for your mind to fully comprehend, and it often feels like you're living in a dream-like state. The shock of loss can make it seem as if you're going through the motions of life on autopilot, and not fully present because it's too damn painful to be.

If none of your peers have experienced grief yet, it's highly likely they'll struggle to fully understand what you're going through. It's almost impossible to put the emotional and physical enormity of loss into words, and when people can't understand the pain you're in, relating to others can be tough.

Feeling 'meh' about life is another common experience after a big loss. You may even have moments of existential crisis where you question the meaning of it all. *What's the point of my life now that my person is no longer here?* It's common to lose interest in activities that you once enjoyed, or find that you aren't as engaged in your relationships as you once were. Trivial or materialistic things can become meaningless – it's not uncommon to feel apathetic, too. You may even go through a period of feeling numb and wonder why you aren't feeling disabling pain. This is all normal. It's not because you don't care, you just don't have the capacity to feel right now, and that's okay.

Grief can also make you feel like a completely different person, impacting your self-esteem and identity. How can you connect with others when you don't even recognise yourself? You might have once been a social butterfly, but now feel a lack of confidence in social situations. It can be hard to explain to people the ways in which grief can reupholster the very fabric of your being, so instead, you might disengage and let relationships fade away.

When we spoke to psychotherapist, author and grief expert Megan Devine, she shared an interesting perspective on why our self-confidence and self-esteem takes such a hit after loss. We are relational beings, she explained. So, when someone you love dies, it's as if you lose both your mirror and your reflection. You stop being able to see yourself clearly because you don't have that relational way of understanding yourself anymore. Without that reverb, you can start to question everything. On top of this, she explains, because grief isn't openly talked about in Western culture, a lot of the outside world says that you are doing grief 'wrong', which causes self-doubt. Not knowing who you are anymore is not doing grief wrong. It's a very normal part of loss. Think about it – you lost somebody who helped you make sense of yourself and the world. Without them, of course it's hard.

You might not even realise that you're feeling disconnected and lonely, but it can show up as feeling pessimistic, self-conscious, spending a lot of time ruminating, filling a void by buying lots of crap you don't need, or avoiding making plans with others. As we'll explore, being vulnerable and speaking honestly about your experience is a vital part of rebuilding your sense of self and connection to the world after loss.

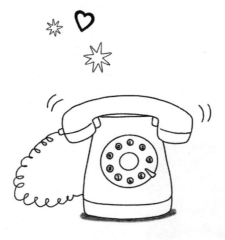

FINDING A LIFELINE

The loneliness of grief caught us both off guard. We consider ourselves well supported, and even though we had friends and family members around us, we still felt lonely in our circumstances.

Living in the same city but unknown to each other, we both searched for online grief support, which led us to an organisation called Motherless Daughters Australia and its private Facebook support group. We didn't realise it then, but a chance meet-up organised by one of the group members would have a big impact on our lives. We both clicked 'attend' on the event, but almost backed out at the eleventh hour. It was nerve-racking to put ourselves out there, especially as we felt so vulnerable and raw in our grief.

Despite our hesitation, we felt a pull to go. Showing up at the pub that day, even though it was completely out of our comfort zones, changed our lives forever. We can both still clearly picture sitting across the table from one another, as each of the ten women attending shared their stories. When each of us took our turn, we felt a connection. You know that feeling when you can just tell someone is your kind of person?

Although we shared a brief overview of our loss, we didn't get a chance to talk properly, or swap numbers. Yet we both had a sense that we would understand what the other person was going through. We thought about each other that evening and, with a bit of courage, a connection was made via Facebook . . .

Hi Sally, it was lovely to meet you yesterday. Although we didn't get a chance to chat one on one, I wanted to reach out as I know we both lost our mums suddenly, and we are similar ages, so I totally know how you must be feeling. Both recently, too. 😞 None of my close friends have lost their mum, so although I have great support, it's still not the same. Here if you ever want someone to chat with, or go over how you're feeling and how unfair it is etc . . . ✨

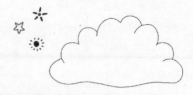

Hi Imogen, it's so lovely to hear from you – thank you so much for your message. I have been meaning to reach out to you to say the same thing actually! I know exactly what you mean about friends being a support but not really knowing what it is like. If you're free in the coming weeks and fancy meeting for a wine and a chat somewhere in the city I'd love that. xx

We arranged to meet and, when we did, we hit it off straight away. We'd finally found a fellow motherless daughter who could understand exactly what we were going through.

In the months that followed, we would meet up and spend hours talking about the world of grief we found ourselves in. We no longer had to pretend that we were doing okay. There were zero platitudes. No uncomfortable small talk. We met each other in our pain and even finished each other's sentences at times. It was like sitting in front of a mirror and having all our griefy thoughts and feelings validated for the first time.

We talked about how lonely we felt and how, at times, like we were losing our minds. One thing we kept coming back to when we'd meet was how little our society talks about grief and how isolating that feels. Here we were, navigating something that is as old as time, yet when we mentioned it, people would stay silent. We wondered how many others were out there, feeling lonely in their grief, just like we were.

One afternoon we had a lightbulb moment – let's start a podcast! And that was the exact moment that Good Mourning was born – a platform to talk candidly about the realities of grief – grief bombs and all. Our mission from the start was to help others feel less alone by talking honestly about loss, just like we did during our meet-ups. We had no idea at the time that we were about to open a door to tens of thousands of other grievers across the world, all looking for the very same things that we were before we met – connection and comfort.

What our community said about . . .

GRIEF AND LONELINESS

'I often feel that people just can't relate, through no fault of their own, but that makes it lonely.'

'My confidence has gone, which means I don't interact with others as much.'

'I can't engage with the world around me. I am on another planet – Planet Grief.'

'I feel like the people around me can't handle my grief and I don't want to exhaust them with it, so I feel isolated.'

'I feel like it's hard to connect with my husband. It's as if I lost part of who I am when my mum died.'

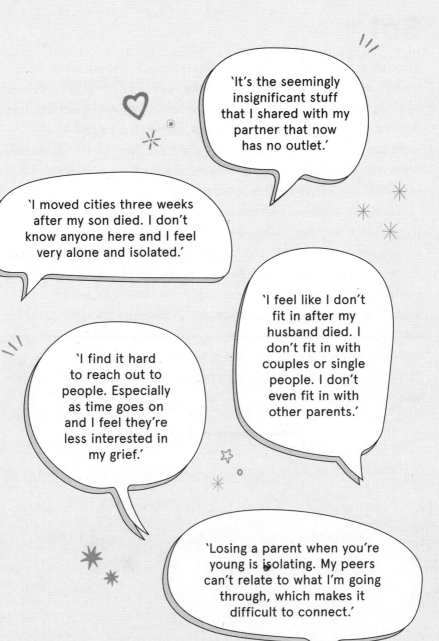

Sal

Being an expat in Australia, most of my support network of family and friends are in the UK. The time of my mum's death also coincided with me moving to a new area where I only knew one person, and a lot of my expat friends moving back home. The people I relied on were distant from me geographically, and because of the pandemic, I was also in lockdown – so seeing them wasn't even an option! This massively contributed to my feelings of loneliness.

Losing Mum made me not only realise how important it is to have a community around you where you physically are, but also to keep in close contact with family and friends back home. For expats, grieving from a distance to those who are also impacted by the loss, and being unable to receive an in-person hug from those closest to you, or share memories about your loved one in person, is tough. Consider setting up a WhatsApp group chat where you can all share your grief and memories. It's also good to schedule in regular video calls. Life can get busy, but it's important to remain connected, especially when you're grieving.

IT'S NORMAL TO

feel lonely

IN GRIEF
(A LITTLE OR A LOT).

IT'S FINE IF YOU
ONLY HAVE A SMALL

support network.

IT'S OKAY IF YOU
HAVE SUPPORT AND

still feel lonely.

Psychologist Tamara's view on coping with loneliness

Social support in grief is necessary because human beings need companionship. We are social creatures, and our relationships give life meaning. It's important that at times you break through your loneliness by reaching out to others and letting them support you. Share how you are feeling with someone you trust, allow them to distract you, or sometimes it can help to simply be in the same physical presence without interacting. This will take time, and I encourage people to be kind to themselves as they navigate a new normal.

Give yourself permission to prioritise your own needs over others' needs at this time. Remind yourself that you can always leave an event early, and plan for flexibility, perhaps by driving yourself to allow for the opportunity to change plans.

If you are feeling like you have no support at all and are experiencing intense loneliness, this may be a time to seek out people who are in a similar situation to you – people who are more likely to be compassionate and understanding of your loss. There are both in-person and online support groups for bereavement and you may find reaching out to one of these helpful. These can include social media groups. Support groups can be especially helpful if you need to reach out to someone currently going through grief and to share day-to-day experiences that resonate. It may also be a time to develop new relationships. You may feel forever changed by your loss and so taking up new activities or cultivating new friendships may help with the feelings of loneliness.

ALONE VS LONELY — WHAT'S THE DIFFERENCE?

There can be an assumption that feeling lonely means a complete absence of others around, but that's not the case. Loneliness is the absence of close connections that meet your social or interpersonal needs, whereas being alone is being physically by yourself. According to mental health professional Eleanor Haley in her article, 'The Unique Loneliness of Grief', loneliness is 'defined by what a person wants in relation to what they have'. Eleanor explains that even if you have lots of friends and family members, if you're longing for something or someone you don't have, such as a spouse you can share intimate moments with, or a parent to confide in, then you're likely to feel lonely.

LONELINESS AND FRIENDSHIPS

Often, we go through *everything* with our friends, and they're our go-to when life goes pear-shaped, offering support and a shoulder to lean on. Except, that's not always the case. As we've discussed, relationships, especially friendships, can shift after a loss. And that's bloody hard, because our friends play such an important role in navigating life's tough challenges.

If your friends or support network haven't experienced loss, they may want to be there for you, but just don't know how. Others might text you the typical 'here for you' sentiments, but not follow through, or they may even completely ghost you (which really f*cking sucks). Others could struggle to provide emotional support and can come across as if they don't care, even though they probably do. Whatever the circumstances, if you can't express or share your grief with your mates, it's a lonely feeling.

Reframing friendships

Not all your friends are going to be able to truly level with you and your loss, but it doesn't mean you can't still have a relationship with them. No matter your age, it's important to understand that everyone plays a different role in your life – accepting that can be key to reframing how you seek support.

Prior to your loss, you may not have even considered that there can be different categories of friends. Greek philosopher Aristotle identified three types: friends of virtue, friends of utility and friends of pleasure. It can be helpful to categorise your friendships by thinking of the three types as different 'buckets'. This exercise can apply to any type of relationship, but because they are often the bedrock of grief support, let's focus on friends.

THE RIDE OR DIES (AKA 'FRIENDS OF VIRTUE')

These are the friends who show up when the going gets tough. These relationships usually take a long time to build, and are few and far between. These people will turn up to your house in the middle of the night if you need them, they're the ones who will sit front row at the funeral and hold your snotty tissues for you.

THE CONVENIENT ONES (AKA 'FRIENDS OF UTILITY')

These are the ones who you only really speak to when you need something (and vice versa). You probably wouldn't call them when you're having a meltdown, but if you need a recommendation for a probate lawyer, they'd be the first on the list.

THE GOOD TIMERS (AKA 'FRIENDS OF PLEASURE')

These are the people you can rely on for a cracking time, but perhaps not for emotional support. These friendships may feel more surface level – perhaps you go out for drinks once in a while, or see each other at social events and have a blast, but these people wouldn't be around to scoop you off the floor if you're hit by a grief bomb.

The benefit of thinking about which friends fall into which bucket is that it helps you look at your support circle in a realistic way. Rather than feeling unsupported because you don't have a bus load of friends showing up around the clock, it allows you to prioritise who to invest energy in.

Not every friend is going to be there for you in your grief in the way that you'd hoped, and that's okay because it's not the role they play. For example, your 'utility friends' and your 'pleasure friends' may not be able to show up for you in your grief, but they can still have a place in your life. There may be a day when you're feeling up to a night on the town and you can count on your one friend of pleasure for a good time, but they may not necessarily be your first port of call on a griefy day. If you're navigating changes in friendships or looking for new mates, then this perspective can help identify what kind of qualities you might want to focus on, and the types of people you could create more space for.

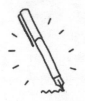

Take a step back and assess who belongs in each friendship 'bucket': the ride or dies, the convenient ones and the good timers. The goal here isn't to cull every person who hasn't stepped up for you in your grief, but to be realistic about your relationships.

Katrina's experience with reframing friendships

'When I was 15, my mum died after being diagnosed with cancer one year earlier. Then, six years later, while I was at university, my baby nephew died from sepsis. Both losses directly impacted my friendships. At the time of Mum's death, none of my peers had lost a parent or significant person in their life and, therefore, they didn't know how to respond. In many cases, they'd remain silent and attempt to ignore the obvious, leading me to feel isolated and alienated. I often felt resentment towards my friends when they'd complain about their mums (as typical teenagers do). While they were out socialising, I was at home attempting to run a household to support my dad. I had to grow up a lot faster than most people my age and found it hard to connect with my peers, so my friendship group remained very small. I had a lot of friends who chose to no longer be in my life because they couldn't cope with my grief and how it had changed me as a person.

'When my nephew died, I was in my final year of university. Yet again, my peers had no understanding of how grief can have a whole-body impact on a person, and a lot of my new friends slowly disappeared. I began abusing alcohol and my friends were unable and unsure how to support me. Some of them didn't want to because I was no longer 'fun' Katrina. I isolated myself from social activities and, consequently, the 'hub' of university life. My perspective of the world, what was important and my responsibilities yet again changed, as did my friendships.'

What helped

'It's 11 years since grief entered my life and I have four friends who have remained and endured all the grief bombs with me. What I've learned is that we have friends for a reason, friends for a season and friends for life. Grief often filters out the first two. Communicating your needs to friends is so important. Don't be afraid to ask for help or share what support you need. People don't leave because there's something wrong with you. Grief doesn't make you broken or unlovable – friendships will change when you experience significant loss because your values change. You're allowed to walk away from people who no longer align with you.'

LONELINESS IN WIDOWHOOD

Losing a partner or spouse is one of the most difficult and distressing experiences we can expect to go through in adult life. So much of your life changes and its very infrastructure, along with your sense of identity, can flip in an instant. A huge factor in loneliness after a life partner or companion dies is that not only do you go from being a duo to single but, even with a social circle, there is no-one else to fulfil their role. You've gone from a team of two to a team of one and the person who knew you like no other is gone. The loss can be very acutely felt through the absence of a shared routine, shared language, physical touch, or having someone to simply do nothing with. Absolutely everything can feel like a trigger when your partner dies – it's unfair, it's overwhelming and it's incredibly isolating.

Psychologist Dr Lauren Breen explained in an *ABC Everyday* article about widowhood that 'loneliness can be compounded by the unexpected judgement of others – with young widows sometimes evoking feelings of fear or even anger in outsiders'. In some cases, you may feel rejected by your coupled friends, and you may find that people withdraw from spending time with you when your partner dies, which can exacerbate your feelings of loneliness. Your partner might have been the glue that connected you to friends and family members, or maybe they were your main form of support and connection. Even if you are a part of a thriving social group, there's a massive void when it comes to doing the mundane, yet intimate, shared things.

While other family members might be grieving, losing a partner can feel like a unique bereavement. Left with the empty bed, the quiet house and the gap of companionship, it can feel like you're starting life all over again. Plus, you might be doing everything solo, learning new things for the first time and taking on new roles and responsibilities that you shared with your other half. Low self-esteem and loss of identity are common – faced with the death of a life partner, you're a shell of yourself and completely discombobulated.

If you're unsure of what steps to take to move forwards, this list might help in easing isolation and rebuilding your self-esteem.

- Give yourself permission to not have it all figured out right now. You have a lot on your plate, and it's okay if you don't know all the answers.
- You might not feel like you've 'got' *any* of this, and no-one expects you to have. Don't be afraid to ask for help. If there are people who want to support you, let them.
- Sometimes, grief makes us do wild things that might not be rational. Selling up and moving to the Bahamas? Sounds like a great plan! Except . . . maybe it's not. Consider getting a

professional opinion before making any big decisions, or even hold off making any for a while.

- Talk to yourself like a friend. Learning new things and taking on new roles isn't easy – it's frustrating, it's hard and you might want to throw in the towel. Give yourself a ton of grace.
- Focus on the relationships with people who give you the space to talk about your feelings. It's okay to distance yourself from those who aren't helping right now.

David's experience with loneliness as a widower

'My wife Bev died in 2016, 14 months after her cancer diagnosis. We'd been together for 13 years and married for almost 11 and during that time our lives became intertwined. I had transitioned from an "I" to a "we" during our time together, and when Bev died, I lost part of me. I now had to figure out how to become an "I" again and what that "I" was now going to look like.

'Those who haven't experienced the death of their person can't understand the depth of the solitude that's at the core of loneliness in widowhood. I had friends and my young son lived at home. Yet, there were many times when I was in a room full of people and still felt like the loneliest person in the world. It was the loneliness that comes with no longer having the person who just "gets" you, from the absence of the everyday interactions with your person that you take for granted.' ⟶

What helped

◁

'Connecting via online support groups to other people who had lost their partners really helped me because they understood my situation. Some online interactions turned into in-person meetings and from that, friendships formed – finding "my tribe" was a big help for me in my grief.'

DISENFRANCHISED GRIEF

Some types of meaningful losses aren't openly acknowledged or even accepted as 'grief worthy' by society. Researcher Kenneth Doka coined the term 'disenfranchised grief' (also known as 'hidden grief'), which includes:

- **non-death losses** – a divorce, loss of health, loss of a job, loss of a home, end of a friendship, romantic break-up, infertility, an absent parent, distancing from toxic family members, a loved one with Alzheimer's or dementia, or a loved one with addiction issues
- **unrecognised relationships** – death of an ex-partner, friend, co-worker, estranged or extended family member, or the death of a pet
- **stigmatised cause of death** – stillborn birth, abortion, miscarriage, suicide, overdose, addiction or homicide.

These types of losses are often minimised or misunderstood by others and can heighten existing feelings of loneliness and isolation. If you've identified with any of these losses, please know that your loss is valid and deserves to be supported. Talk therapy and support groups can provide a safe and supportive space where you can discuss your feelings and feel understood as you begin to process your grief. We've included a bunch of supportive resources and organisations on pages 289–92, which you may find helpful.

Im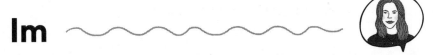

People don't know how to respond to death at the best of times, but when it comes to a death by suicide, people *really* don't know what to say. The sense of shock relating to my mum's death was incredibly isolating. I felt like no-one understood the complicated pain I was feeling. When strangers asked how my mum died, I wouldn't even know where to begin for fear of their judgement. It's not uncommon for people to find it difficult to confide in others and even avoid telling them the cause of death. There's unfortunately still a stigma that's attached to suicide, which contributes to feelings of shame, loneliness and social isolation.

There are a lot of preconceived notions about suicide and one of them is that suicide only affects people with mental illness. This isn't true. My mum had no pre-existing mental health conditions. She was going through an unimaginably traumatic event in her life and was experiencing what's called 'situational depression'.

Because I felt that very few people could understand the complexity of what I was experiencing, I found strength in connecting with other suicide loss survivors. Allianceofhope.org is a fantastic resource for anyone coping with suicide loss. They have a forum that operates like a 24/7 support group, where you can read other people's experiences, share your own, and connect with people who understand exactly what you're going through.

What our community said about . . .

DISENFRANCHISED GRIEF

'I had a miscarriage when I was 20 years old. Everyone told me I was way too young for a child anyway; I was heartbroken.'

'I am chronically ill and have an invisible disability, but people don't understand that my whole life has changed, and I am unable to do the things I want to do. I am grieving, but it's not recognised as "traditional grief", so it's ignored and misunderstood.'

'I left my husband because of his alcohol addiction, and he died five months later. I feel lonely, sad, heartbroken, and like I don't deserve to be grieving because we weren't together anymore.'

'My ex-partner died of stomach cancer. We were best friends. No-one ever talks to me about it, and I feel invisible.'

'I have an abusive parent with whom I have chosen not to have contact, for the sake of my mental health. People don't understand how painful it is to grieve someone who is still alive, but with whom you aren't able to have a relationship.'

'My best friend died, and I feel like because I wasn't family, my grief isn't important.'

'My estranged dad died six weeks after my mum, and no-one ever acknowledges his death.'

'I am grieving the loss of my therapist who died. I'd been seeing her for seven years, through my divorce and the loss of my mum. I am devastated. I feel like no-one understands and I don't have anyone to talk to about it.'

'My brother died by suicide and it's as if everyone is scared that grief's contagious, and their loved ones will die if they acknowledge it, so nobody brings it up.'

THE IMPORTANCE OF CONNECTION

When you're feeling lonely and disconnected from others, the natural tendency is to withdraw. In an article on their website called 'How to Overcome Loneliness', Self Space, a therapy service, explains that when we feel emotionally vulnerable, it can make us view our existing relationships in a negative light, believing the people around us care much less than they actually do. We might worry that people don't want to hear about our loss, or might not understand, and so we hesitate to reach out. It can be a bit of a self-fulfilling prophecy, meaning that if we think people aren't interested in supporting us, we continue to feel isolated. And loneliness becomes a cycle that can be difficult to break.

Everyone craves connection, no matter how independent you are, or how comfortable you are in your own company. Why? Because it's key to easing feelings of loneliness. When you feel like you have someone who 'gets' you and your grief, you're more likely to authentically express yourself and feel truly seen, heard and supported. And right now, you need and deserve all of that.

To get through loss we need great people by our side, and it all starts with building a solid foundation, that is made up of the following:

COMMUNICATION

A big part of building intimacy in relationships comes from communicating well. You need to be able to listen to someone and tell them how you feel, and vice versa. The more you feel like you understand them and they understand you, the closer your connection becomes.

TRUST

Trusting others with your emotions might not always be easy, but it's worth it because you must be able to trust others to foster intimacy.

When you're choosing someone to develop stronger and deeper bonds with, make sure it's someone you feel you can trust. In turn, you need to show them that they can trust you. Trust is a two-way street.

CURIOSITY

Nothing builds intimacy more than feeling like others know what makes you tick. A good way to establish deeper bonds is to ask questions and make an effort to learn about others. Dig deeper than surface level and try to really get to know them. In turn, they'll hopefully do the same for you. When you ask questions, make sure you listen, so you can develop a true understanding of the other person, and what makes them tick, too.

APPRECIATION

Showing people that you appreciate them can go a long way to building connections. Thank them for the things they do. Take time to do something nice for them out of the blue, such as buying them their favourite snacks, writing a thoughtful note to them or cooking them a meal you know they enjoy.

EMPATHY

Being empathetic to others and showing emotional connections can help you form deeper relationships. It shows that you really understand and relate to others, and that can be a great way to create intimacy, trust and belonging.

Developing closer connections isn't something that's instantaneous. You won't share a deep feeling or secret with someone and instantly score 100 per cent on an intimacy test. However, if you keep trying, you might just see that developing deeper connections eases loneliness.

Once a day, at least, commit to connecting with a friend, family member, colleague or someone in the online community via text, email or a call. Set a reminder if you need to, and make it a part of your day. Try organising a video call with a friend or, if you're looking to meet like-minded people, joining a grief support group (online or in person), signing up for a class, taking up a new hobby or volunteering in your community.

Got someone in mind you want to connect with? Here are some conversation starters for when you're not feeling yourself.

- 'Hey! I would love to see you more often. Can we organise a catch-up?'
- 'I want to let you know how much your support has meant to me. I am still having a difficult time, but knowing you are there helps me immensely. Can we meet for a coffee sometime soon?'
- 'You are such a valued friend to me, and your support means so much to me during this time. Talking to you has really helped. Are you free for me to call you this week?'
- 'I'd really like to see you more often. How do you feel about making our meet-ups more regular?'

 Don't be afraid of a little solitude. It's okay to be alone sometimes and it doesn't mean that there's anything wrong with you. Try seeing alone time as an opportunity to reflect on how you're feeling and what you need to take the next step forwards (just make sure you balance it with spending some time with others).

Glenda's experience with reaching out

'My dearest friend, Helen, died two years after being diagnosed with cancer. She was only 52. Without Helen, I would not have survived my dad's death ten years earlier – she climbed down into my "grief pit" and offered me constant support.

'I find Helen's absence and the loneliness of grief excruciating. When I felt the most alone in my grief, I would also start to doubt what else I was feeling. To navigate this, I tended to spiral into toxic positivity – I would think I should be grateful for the life that I have, I should be grateful to be alive, that life could be so much worse and that it would be so much harder if I was in Helen's family. At one point, I concluded that the solution was to never allow myself to form another deep connection again. This was completely irrational because I know that, for me, connection is what makes life worthwhile.'

What helped

'Finding the courage to discuss my grief and how I was feeling has been helpful. When I made the effort to reach out and connect to others, people who loved and cared about me would engage and did want to listen. Most of them just did not know how to ask questions or whether I wanted to speak about it. I think other people who have experienced the intense loneliness of grief are drawn to you, and you to them, so often when you do reach out you will find someone else who is familiar with that loneliness. The pain is universal and often I have formed deep connections based on that understanding.'

THE POWER OF GRIEF SUPPORT

When you find other people who are going through loss, it can make a world of difference. Grief support can be a game-changer when you're feeling lonely, disconnected and like no-one understands. As we've discussed, connecting with others who have experienced loss can help you feel seen and heard. What we love about grief support is that it offers a safe space for you to share your story or experience in an environment free from judgement. There can be a HUGE sense of relief when you find people who understand. Like our experience when we met, there's no need to pretend you're okay or gloss over your emotions.

We spoke to authors Ellidy Pullin and Lotte Bowser about their experience connecting through social media after their partners, Alex and Ben, both died in their 30s. For Ellidy and Lotte, being widowed at a young age was incredibly isolating. They explained how finding each other, and sharing their experiences of being young and widowed, saved them both during an unimaginably difficult time.

Grief support also provides a space to learn more about the grief process and coping strategies – we love it when we hear from our podcast listeners and online community that something we've said or shared has helped them better understand what they're going through. The type of support you seek is up to you. You can focus on your specific type of loss, like we did through Motherless Daughters Australia. Or if you are dealing with loneliness after the death of your spouse, it might make sense to join a support group for widows and widowers. There are lots of general grief support groups out there to join (such as our free private Facebook group, Good Mourning Grief Support Group) that can be a great source of comfort, understanding and connection, no matter your loss. We've witnessed many friendships formed over shared experiences in the comments.

Before you attend a support group, whether that's in-person or online, be prepared for your emotions to come to the surface when you're talking about your loss or hearing the stories of others. Expressing your grief can be confronting, especially if you haven't had a lot of support. It may also be the first time you've connected with other grievers, and you may be surprised at how others share their grief, or respond to the group, so remember that we all grieve differently and on different timelines. Grief support groups are different from counselling or therapy – if you're struggling with feelings of loneliness, we always recommend that you speak to a therapist.

HERE ARE SOME EXCELLENT GRIEF ACCOUNTS TO CONNECT WITH ON INSTAGRAM

@goodmourningpodcast (obviously!)

@griefkid

@grieflineorganisation

@lifedeathwhat

@marklemonofficial

@modernloss

@refugeingrief

@talkaboutloss

@thebiggrief

@thedinnerparty

@thegriefcase

@thegriefgangpodcast

@untanglegrief

@whatsyourgrief

It's great to use social media to find grief support, but be mindful about how you are using it. If you find that going online and looking at what others are up to is making you feel worse, it's a good idea to either limit your use or take a break.

Leda's experience with finding grief support

'I lost my son Marlowe during birth in January 2021. Never did I think something like this would happen to me and I was plunged into a world of dark grief. No-one I knew had ever experienced a loss like this – it's very different from losing a parent or a friend. I had tons of support from friends and family, but I still felt incredibly alone. There was no-one who could quite understand my unique pain – not even my loving husband. My mind was reeling in pain at the future I'd planned for and my body was physically grieving the loss of not being able to nurture my baby. Many mornings I would wake up in a state of panic thinking, *What do I do now?*

'I knew I had to find other women to connect to who could speak the same heartbroken language as me. A social worker's name was passed to me and she connected me to a woman who had experienced the same hell as me. The instant we met, we hugged and said, "Okay, who wants to go first?", referring to showing a photo of our little lost loves. She was my immediate friend and I didn't want to leave her presence. She understood me. She "got" me.'

What helped

'I joined a support group that was set up by the hospital. I was incredibly nervous, angry and even shameful walking into my first session. I didn't want to be there. It felt weird; I was meant to be in a mothers' group talking about baby things and complaining joyfully about my lack of sleep! It was confronting and comforting all at the same time. I wasn't alone – I was far from alone. It was there that I bonded with two women who I know I can call day or night and they will be at the end of the line listening to me. Without my support friends, the days would have been much longer and much darker. As humans, we need to find our community. I know I'm in a much better headspace because I found "my people".'

Nama's experience with finding support outside of her family

'When I got the call that my sister had died at 42, my first thought was, *I'll never speak to her again.* My second thought was for my mother and that she wouldn't ever recover from this, having lost my father a few years earlier. I knew that I couldn't burden my broken mum with my own grief, so I made the decision to not share the depths of my grief with anyone, except for my other two sisters, who were just as devastated as I was. →

◁ 'The three of us quickly discovered that we were at different stages of processing our grief at various times. Supporting each other in grief is a lot about timing – and being on the same timeline. I learned to be careful about just calling up and bursting into tears, as I so often wanted to do, lest I disturb any hard-won peace for them at that moment. I shared my grief with my sisters, but I tried to walk the fine line of not burdening them, too. That's what led me to online grief groups. I realised that anyone active in the group at the time I went in there was prepared to listen and support. If they weren't, they didn't have to engage. With online grief support groups, timing wasn't an issue – people were there to help. Strangers wanted to help, empathise and make my grief feel less isolating.'

What helped

'Hearing the experiences of others helped me. I found that I could even offer some advice to those who had lost a parent or a sibling and that also gave me a sense of purpose. My advice is don't be afraid to seek out a grief support group – they offer a unique community you can rely on, even though it's one no-one wants to be in.'

What our community said about . . .

FINDING GRIEF SUPPORT

'I love that everyone is able to express their authentic feelings, with no judgement.'

'I feel less alone and my thoughts and emotions are validated.'

'Being part of a community makes me feel understood.'

'I just love knowing that there are others out there who understand what grief is really like.'

'Being able to connect with people in a similar situation, for me, is community therapy.'

'The support from a group helped me validate my feelings, because I can see that others are experiencing them, too.'

'It helps me learn about my grief so I can understand it better.'

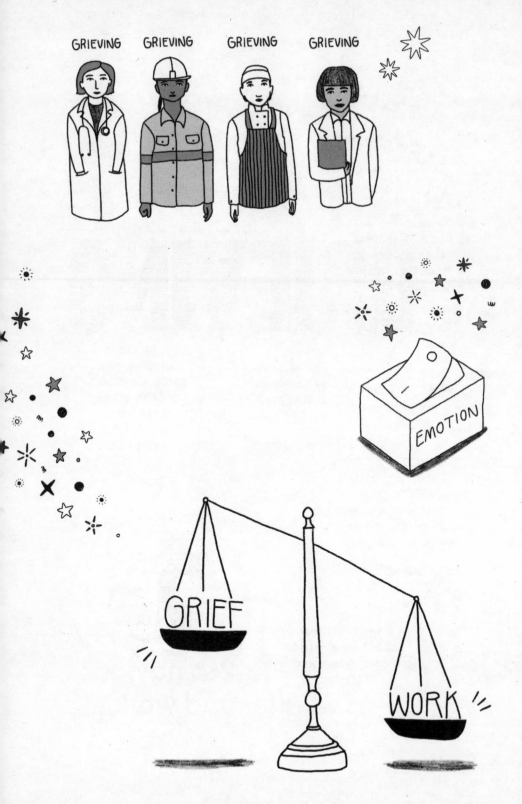

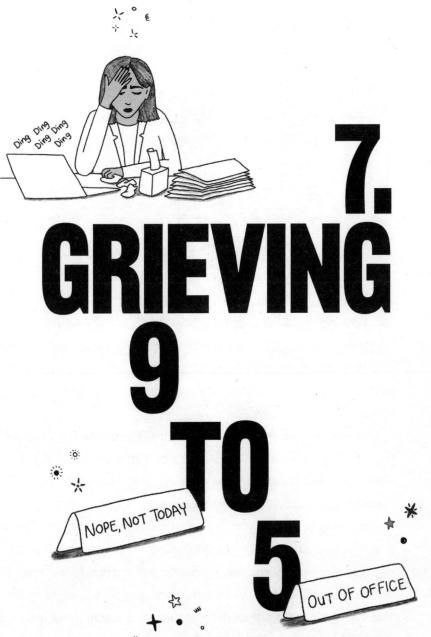

7.
GRIEVING
9 TO 5

NOPE, NOT TODAY

OUT OF OFFICE

How to navigate grief and work

GOING BACK TO WORK AFTER A LOSS CAN FEEL SURREAL.

Although it's often invisible to your colleagues, grief isn't absent from the working day. Whatever your profession, it's always lurking in the background. It's there when you're in meetings, serving customers or checking emails. A grief bomb can hit unexpectedly and then – *WHAM!* – the floodgates open. Although it's nothing to be ashamed of, ugly crying at work can be mortifying.

When you're emotionally and physically exhausted, it's not easy to push your grief aside to face a full day on the job. As we discussed in Chapter 3, the emotional stress of grief can feel debilitating and impact concentration, confidence and motivation.

The level of empathy and support from co-workers can play a big part in how well you cope – or don't cope – with grief at work. Life has changed irrevocably and small talk, or minor complaints, feel trivial. You're going through a monumental experience, talking to colleagues about an issue that's urgent to them, but feels unimportant to you. *Who cares if the printer is broken? My person is dead!* you scream internally.

Whether you're transitioning back to work after loss, or you've been balancing grief and work for a while, it's only natural that grief will pop up at work. After all, you're dealing with one of life's biggest challenges. Be gentle with yourself and remember, what you're going through right now is super tough and you are doing the best you can. You can't always escape the 9-to-5 grind, but there are ways to help you get through it.

RETURNING TO WORK WHEN YOU'RE GRIEVING

As much as you might want to take off a long period of time after a loss, in reality, it's not always possible. Short bereavement leave or financial pressures could see you returning to work sooner than you feel ready. It's common to feel that you didn't have enough time to even process the death, let alone start to properly grieve. The thought of going back to work can be overwhelming for some, but on the flip side, work can be a lifeline to others – having a sense of routine and normality can be reasons to want to get back to it, pronto.

A big factor in navigating grief and work is how people respond to your loss. Some might offer great support and show empathy, while others could be awkward or not acknowledge it at all, which can be incredibly uncomfortable. When the office chat is along the lines of, 'Hey! How are you?', 'Great, thanks!' can be an easy reply to manage the risk of breaking down. Talking about death can make some people feel scared to do or say the wrong thing, especially if they haven't experienced a loss. So, if you feel able to, it can be a good idea to write a short note (or email) to your co-workers to let them know what they can do to support you.

No matter how long you were able to take off work, the transition period back can be hard, especially if you're feeling like it's difficult to get your work done at the same pace. It's important to ensure you get all the help that you can, so ask your employer if they have an employee assistance program (EAP), which can provide support and access to counselling and other health services. If they don't, you might need to be more direct in asking for what you need, such as flexibility to attend appointments, or shorter working hours to give you some space to breathe and to process your loss.

Camilla's experience with going back to work

'In 2013 we lost our triplet girls. Elina was stillborn, Signe died after eight days and Ines died after seven weeks. My whole pregnancy was a difficult one and was high risk, so I was basically on sick leave from day one after the positive pregnancy test. As an ambitious teacher, I found that hard, but I was also worried about what would happen to my three babies.

'During my pregnancy, my principal wanted me to visit whenever I had the strength, so I went to work on a couple of Wednesdays. After the girls were all born extremely premature, we ended up in the hospital and I began a new period of sick leave. Those weeks of caring for very fragile babies took its toll. When we finally lost Ines, going back to work felt far, far away. We struggled to get up every morning, but we had to – we had our son to take care of.

'We lost Ines in October, and by January, I felt it was time to go back to work again. However, going back to my class of 28 children was out of the question, and working full-time? A big no-no! My boss simply said to me, "Listen, Camilla, we will find you something to do, something that you feel you can handle. All that's important is that you are here. You'll work

50 per cent and we'll take it from there." I could hardly believe how much compassion he showed, and that was the turning point for me feeling ready to go back to work.'

What helped

'Seeing a psychologist helped me prepare to go back to work. She gave me coping tools, which made the transition easier.'

~~~~~~~~

Lisa's experience with taking extra time off

'One morning, I missed a call from my sister. Even though it was early, it was not early enough for me to worry. I called her back, and she said, "I have to tell you something hard . . . Mum didn't wake up this morning." It's right on a year since that phone call, and I am still reeling with not just grief, but the immense shock.

'The timing of Mum's sudden death came at a very complicated time (as if any time is better or worse for something like that). I was experiencing severe burnout from taking care of my toddler while trying to work from home. I had worked up the courage to ask for a six-week sabbatical from work that had started five weeks before Mum's sudden death, with only one more week left of the six weeks. I took a deep breath and asked for my sabbatical to be extended to another three weeks. It was granted and I was relieved.'→

What helped

'I decided to be honest about what I needed and not be afraid to share my grief with others, or express the impact that Mum's sudden death had on me.'

WORKING AND WEEPING

You're probably going to have days when it's hard to motor through – there might even be days where you are physically present, but your mind isn't. Instead of focusing on the task at hand, you're probably preoccupied with thoughts about your person or worries about the future. It can be bloody hard to keep it together for eight consecutive hours (or more) in a work environment. You might be trying your best to muddle through the day, fighting back the sadness, shock, tears and general fatigue, unsure if what you're experiencing is normal. Perhaps you're finding it hard to concentrate or digest information.

Working at the same pace as before can feel impossible, and your enthusiasm might have plummeted. We talked about brain fog or 'grief brain' in Chapter 3, and it often shows up at work. The stress of simply trying to survive grief can impact your cognitive function. You may feel an expectation from colleagues to be back to your normal, high-functioning self, which can send you into a spiral of self-doubt. Grief impacts the things that help you to perform well – focus, memory recall, processing information and making judgement calls. It's important to know that if you aren't able to function as well at work, it's not a reflection of your ability – it's a normal response to loss.

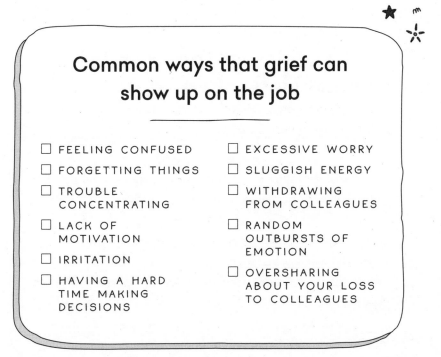

Common ways that grief can show up on the job

- [ ] FEELING CONFUSED
- [ ] FORGETTING THINGS
- [ ] TROUBLE CONCENTRATING
- [ ] LACK OF MOTIVATION
- [ ] IRRITATION
- [ ] HAVING A HARD TIME MAKING DECISIONS
- [ ] EXCESSIVE WORRY
- [ ] SLUGGISH ENERGY
- [ ] WITHDRAWING FROM COLLEAGUES
- [ ] RANDOM OUTBURSTS OF EMOTION
- [ ] OVERSHARING ABOUT YOUR LOSS TO COLLEAGUES

If you've ticked off any of the above, know that it's normal and that the brain fog will ease over time. As you navigate it, give yourself a truckload of self-compassion. A good way to tackle the overwhelm is to break your day into chunks and diarise your tasks. This way, you can see in your work calendar what you can realistically get done. If you are working at a slower pace, remember to give yourself a little more time than you think you need to digest information. The aim here is not to put any undue pressure on yourself. Also, when you feel forgetful, sticky notes are a godsend. Write down everything that needs to get done and stick them around you.

And remember, if things don't make much sense or you're forgetful and confused, understand that it does not mean that you're failing. It just means that you're *grieving*.

Psychologist Tamara's view on coping with grief at work

Many people worry that they will unexpectedly be tearful or unable to cope. If you feel overwhelmed, distraction can help and there are many short-term grounding techniques that you can use. But ultimately, remind yourself that it's okay to grieve. Be upset if you need and never apologise for being upset when it's perfectly expected given your loss.

If you have leave available, use it to its fullest extent. This means avoiding checking emails or making phone calls, and creating a clear boundary between you and your employer that gives you proper time to utilise your leave. If you're unable to take time off but it's possible for you to work from home or work more flexible hours, then discuss this with your manager.

If you have a less understanding workplace, it may be very difficult to juggle your work commitments while processing your grief. Expect to have greater trouble concentrating, lack motivation, be forgetful and be at an increased risk of illness or injury during this time. There is no shame in saying no to additional work or asking your manager to lighten your work duties temporarily.

While you're under no obligation to share details of your grief with colleagues, some people do find this beneficial. You may give permission for your manager to disclose this to colleagues via email, or choose to speak to people yourself. Keep in mind that many of your colleagues will be well-meaning, even if it appears they are not. If some seem distant or unconcerned, they may be uncomfortable with grief themselves, and you are not responsible for their discomfort.

Kayleigh's experience with being open about grief at work

'My dad died of cancer at 57. I'd been in my job for three years, barely taking a day off for sickness, but in the weeks leading up to his death, I had to ask for time off to take him to his appointments, operations and scans. Carrying the responsibility of Dad's health and life while maintaining a full-time job was hard. My whole life outside of work was consumed with worry about what was going to happen, and work became a bit of an escape.

'No-one at work knew Dad had gone into hospital. I didn't think he'd die, so I didn't tell them. But he did. The next day, work rang me to say that they wanted to send an email out to everyone, "so nobody thinks you've done something wrong". I didn't care. Even now, in a new role, it feels weird to mention the most personal and traumatic thing that has ever happened to me. How do I share that with new people, who didn't know him or our relationship?'

What helped

'I use humour (inappropriately, to some), because I'm so conscious of other people being uncomfortable. It's not as a defence mechanism for me, but for others, to hopefully make them feel comfortable and to know it's okay to talk about it. Whether it's talking to a therapist or writing in a journal, remember that it's all about your own pace and when you feel comfortable to tell people.'

Elizabeth's experience with 'grief brain' at work

'It was a normal Tuesday at work for me with the usual emails, meetings and juggling the new home-schooling life due to a lockdown, but all with the absence of my mum's phone calls due to her being so sick in bed. My workday had finished like every other, but the next time I would log onto the computer would be a week-and-a-half later and everything in my life would have changed. My mum died that afternoon.

'In my first team meeting back after time off, I was delivered a "welcome back, Elizabeth" as if I had returned from an around-the-world trip. I wasn't the same person, and I certainly wasn't the same bubbly team member they knew. I've known my manager for six years and was very open in explaining that I was having issues catching up on work, because I had so much on my mind – work, but also dealing with probate and closing Mum's bank accounts. I was the one doing all the life admin work Mum left behind, ensuring my family was kept in the loop of what was happening (and things happened slowly).

'Despite all this, work kept coming and new projects were given to me. I explained to my boss that I was part-time and was struggling with capacity, but it fell on deaf ears. In their eyes, the work had to be done. I had many breakdowns. One good thing about being home due to lockdowns was that I could cry in private and keep my camera off in meetings. In the end, I had to think of my own mental health and general wellbeing. I stuck to my hours, not doing more or less, and organised my day with tasks that I could get through.'

What helped

'Exercise became an important part of my day. Walking with my son and listening to podcasts kept my mind away from thoughts of Mum dying and what emails would be waiting for me when I returned to my desk.'

It can be helpful to identify the ways that grief is showing up for you during your workday so that you can support yourself as best as possible.

* *Is your grief showing up in specific ways?*
* *Are you finding certain people hard to cope with?*
* *Are there certain tasks that are taking you longer to do?*
* *What areas are you struggling with the most?*
* *Are there any external factors that you're coping with outside of work, such as settling the estate, that you could flag with your boss?*
* *Can you have an honest conversation with your manager about how you are coping?*
* *What two things would you change to help yourself right now?*

HOW TO HAVE YOUR OWN BACK

It makes no difference whether you've got a 'grief saint' of a boss or feel like a tumbleweed blows through the office every time you mention your loss – the one person who can help get you through the workday is you. So, when the grief bombs hit, your to-do list is mounting and you're struggling to concentrate, what can you do to support yourself?

YOUR LOSS, YOUR WAY

If you have the headspace or opportunity, you can have a say in how your employers share your situation with your colleagues. If you don't feel like telling people en masse, it might be worth asking your employer to let the people you work most closely with know about your situation. This might help prevent people from saying anything insensitive, while also helping you feel supported. You have the option to let your employer know how you want your situation to be communicated, and if it's okay to talk about your loss.

ASK FOR FLEXIBILITY

If you need more flexibility, it's worth discussing this with your employer. Maybe it's asking for shorter hours while you adjust, a few days a week working from home, or time out to attend counselling sessions or personal appointments. It's important to know what support is available to you. If you don't know what your options are, your manager or HR department will, so be sure to ask.

YOU CAN HAVE BOUNDARIES

Not everyone feels comfortable having their personal situation shared and that's perfectly fine. You don't have to discuss your situation with anyone other than the people who need to know. If someone asks you about the death, and you don't feel up to explaining, it's okay to establish a boundary by politely telling them you're not in the headspace to talk about it right now.

ESTABLISH A CODE WORD

A good idea for extra-griefy days is establishing a code word with a supportive manager or other colleague who has got your back. If you have to take a break, get out of a meeting, or need some support but don't want to make it obvious, this could be a good plan.

FIND A PROOF PAL

Grief can make concentrating and focusing on fine details difficult to do, which means we might make mistakes. Ask a colleague to double-check important items in your work. It could help you avoid making any big errors, and also give your teammates an extra way to help you.

SEEK OUT A TRUSTED 'SUPER SUPPORTER'

Sometimes, knowing you have someone you can call on throughout the day for support, a cry, a hug or a cup of tea can save the day. Maybe it's your HR manager or a co-worker who would listen to you without any judgement, give you space to talk about your person or sit quietly with you if you need to cry. Whoever it is, make sure it's a person who you feel *completely* comfortable around.

Also, you could ask your HR manager to act as a go-between with other colleagues – things like letting others know how you are doing and what you need, or helping to distribute your workload or tasks if it feels too much.

HAVE AN ESCAPE PLAN

The truth is, there can be heavy days when you're grieving. When they strike, it can be super awkward to explain to others. It's good to have a plan if you feel overwhelmed and need to leave work, without going into detail. Sometimes a supportive silent nod is all that's needed. It's worth having an open conversation with your manager to agree that on heavy days, it's okay to give them the heads up and work from home. Or agreeing that if you do a vanishing act, they'll know it's because you're struggling, and you don't have to explain yourself.

TALK ABOUT YOUR PERSON

Talking about your loved one can be a way to signal to others that you're comfortable discussing your loss and that it's okay to ask about them. A memento or a photo on your desk is a simple way to signal to others that you are open to discussing your loss, which can help you feel supported.

PREPARE FOR IMPORTANT DATES

Milestones like anniversaries and birthdays, plus the days leading up to them, can blindside you with griefy emotions. If you've got a big date coming up and you think that the grief bombs might be hitting hard, plan to take the day off. Schedule a day for a big grief sesh (see page 69), or do something to honour your loved one. Whatever you do, if you can, take leave on or around those dates (more on coping with milestones in Chapter 8).

If you prefer being at work as a distraction during those milestone dates, that's also okay. You could explain to your co-workers what day it is, so they can be ready to support you if you need it.

SET ASIDE SOME TIME FOR SELF-CARE

Working and grieving (even if you are working from home) can be exhausting. So, take time to rest and recharge. Keep your schedule flexible and stressors to the minimum (if you can). This is a great opportunity to add some of those 'micro-rituals' that we talked about in Chapter 4 into your routine, both at work and after work. For example:

- take two minutes to meditate before work.
- drink a cup of your favourite tea.
- prepare a nourishing lunch.
- read a few chapters of a good book.
- call a friend to connect.
- go for a long walk after work.
- listen to calming music on your commute.

WHEN YOU'RE SELF-EMPLOYED

What happens if you're self-employed and in charge of your schedule? You might have a team to take care of, or you might be a solo operator, but either way, running a business or venture of your own can be tiring on top of grief, and you need to make sure you look after yourself properly.

BE HONEST AND OPEN

Grief can make us short, snappy and forgetful. If you have employees, be honest about your situation (if you feel comfortable). If you're absent, irritable or just having a tough day and need a break, people will understand why.

DELEGATE OR OUTSOURCE

If you're struggling, need time off or don't have as much headspace, it's a good idea to delegate some of your tasks. Could someone else take a meeting for you? Could you pass on some admin to another team member?

TAKE REGULAR BREAKS

You are a human, not a machine. Take small breaks to reset throughout the day.

EAT AWAY FROM YOUR DESK

It can be a way to break up the day and create a bit of space for yourself, especially if you're a freelancer working from home.

CREATE AN END-OF-DAY ROUTINE

This is a good way to 'close off' work for the day. Close your laptop and go for a walk, or do some yoga.

BE CONSCIOUS OF 'YOU' TIME

It can be easy when self-employed to work longer hours. Make sure you check-in with yourself and that you're not overdoing it. Give yourself deadlines for when you stop checking business emails for the day so that you allow yourself time to rest.

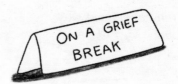

THIS IS YOUR PERMISSION TO

call in

sad

TO WORK IF YOU NEED TO.

Kate's experience with a workmate who understands grief

'In 2009, when I was 13, my father passed away and my mother became my pillar of strength. Twelve years later, in March 2021, she was diagnosed with cancer in multiple organs and died nine weeks later. I was, and still am, devastated. I am a teacher and the school summer holidays started around the time my mum died. I had 12 weeks to learn to cope without her and get my life together, before the new term started.

'As the time to go back to work got closer, I became anxious. My stomach would churn at the thought of the first day of school, seeing people and a big deal being made of me, and I dreaded the questions they would ask. When I did return to work, it wasn't that bad – most of my colleagues and students were immensely supportive and understanding; they understood my need to come in and do my job. Some people did make comments or offered unnecessary advice. After the first day back at work, I received a text message from a colleague with several grief counsellors' numbers.'

What helped

'I work with my best friend, and she became my "grief bouncer". As someone close to me, she knows when I'm having a terrible day and helps me to manage by letting others know it's a tough day, or being mindful of what I take on. I recommend confiding in someone close to you at work so that they can have your back.'

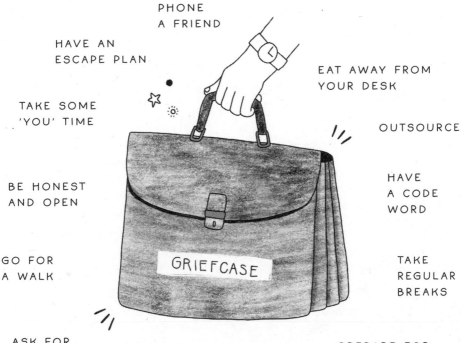

PHONE
A FRIEND

HAVE AN
ESCAPE PLAN

EAT AWAY FROM
YOUR DESK

TAKE SOME
'YOU' TIME

OUTSOURCE

BE HONEST
AND OPEN

HAVE
A CODE
WORD

GO FOR
A WALK

GRIEFCASE

TAKE
REGULAR
BREAKS

ASK FOR
FLEXIBILITY

PREPARE FOR
MILESTONES

FIND A
PROOF PAL

SEEK OUT
A 'SUPER
SUPPORTER'

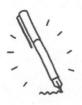

There may be days when you have to show up at work, but your grief feels very heavy. It's good to have a plan in place for these days – let's call it your grief survival kit, aka your 'griefcase'. Based on the tips in this chapter, what might you pack it with to support yourself? Maybe it's a code word, taking regular breaks or adding some self-care into your day?

What our community said about ...

COPING WITH GRIEF AT WORK

'If you're not supported, don't be afraid to look for another job. I quit mine and it was the best thing I did.'

'Let people know your comfort zone and if it's okay for them to talk about your loss or not.'

'Make sure everyone knows. It's a part of your story.'

'Take time out if you need it. Find a person you can talk to on bad days.'

'Answer truthfully if a colleague asks how you are doing. People don't listen, but at least you are being yourself.'

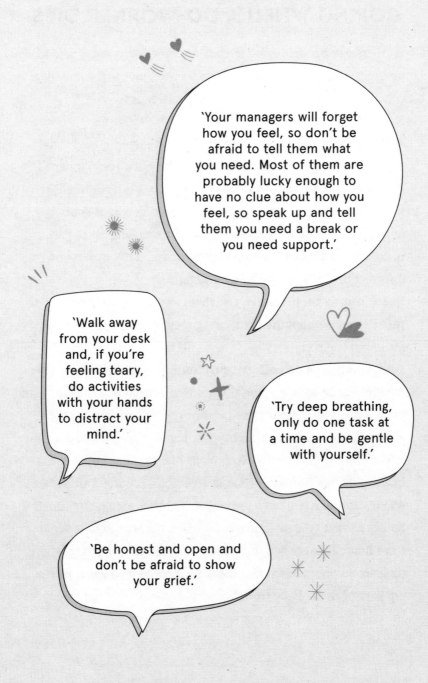

'Your managers will forget how you feel, so don't be afraid to tell them what you need. Most of them are probably lucky enough to have no clue about how you feel, so speak up and tell them you need a break or you need support.'

'Walk away from your desk and, if you're feeling teary, do activities with your hands to distract your mind.'

'Try deep breathing, only do one task at a time and be gentle with yourself.'

'Be honest and open and don't be afraid to show your grief.'

COPING WHEN A CO-WORKER DIES

Co-workers can become good friends and, for some, more like family. If you are mourning the death of a co-worker, here are some ideas on how you can support yourself and your colleagues.

- **Acknowledge your loss as a team.** Don't sweep it under the carpet. Find a time to talk together about what has happened.
- **Establish a team communicator.** If there is a team member who had a close relationship with the person who died, it might make sense for them to be the person who takes care of communication, or acts as a conduit to clarify or pass on information, such as the funeral details.
- **Reach out to their family.** Let them know you are thinking of them. Send a sympathy card, or a practical gift, such as vouchers for a meal delivery service.
- **Do something as a collective to honour their memory.** This could be creating a memorial book that everyone writes in, with photos and memories of the person. It's a good way to talk about the loss and share memories, but also might make a nice gift to send to the family. You might like to organise an event in the person's honour, or name an employee award after them and invite their family to present it. Another idea is inviting the family to visit your workplace. So often our work life is separate from home life, but it can be lovely for the family to see where their loved one worked and meet the people who were such a big part of their 'away from home' life.

MANAGING ANTICIPATORY GRIEF AT WORK

It's not just after a death that you may be feeling griefy at work. Anticipatory grief (which we discussed in Chapter 1) can also impact your work life. It might not always be possible to leave work to care full-time for someone, meaning that you might need to juggle a job *and* being a carer. Knowing that someone is going to die, and having to plan for the goodbye, while holding down employment can be exhausting – emotionally, mentally and physically. It's common to feel hypervigilant if you're waiting for a phone call with bad news, and that can make it hard to focus.

If this sounds like you, then having extra support is vital and preparing colleagues for what's to come is important. Maybe that means having an open conversation with your team so they are clear on what you're dealing with, or making sure there's a plan in place if you do need to take time off at short notice.

Here are some tips for coping with anticipatory grief at work:

- Tell your colleagues about your situation if they don't already know. Depending on your preferences, you might want to ask that they don't ask you about it at work, if it's upsetting. Alternatively, you might prefer that they do check-in, so you feel supported.
- Before the death occurs, ask for clarity on how long you can take off for bereavement leave. This means you will have a clear plan in place. If you anticipate that you'll have to do a lot of the organising with the funeral and estate, it might be worth asking for extra time off.
- Talk to your employer about having a back-up plan in case you need to leave work suddenly. It can be helpful to map out what

your company will tell the team, what the key priorities are that need to be taken care of, and who covers your workload.

- While you're at work, you may feel guilty for not taking care of your person. It might help alleviate some stress to have friends or family members to help shoulder the load while you're at work. That can help give you peace of mind and means you can be regularly updated.

Nikki's experience with anticipatory grief at work

'Mike, my soulmate, was diagnosed with osteosarcoma at the age of 30. Initially, the prognosis was relatively good, with surgery and chemotherapy that took a year. My work during this time was supportive; they gave me the flexibility to work away from the office so I could be with him.

'Mike underwent treatment and, during his final appointment, we were told he was terminal. I called work as we were leaving the hospital to give them the news. That is when the support dropped away – all I got was a reply saying, "Will you not be back in the office this afternoon, then?" The comments and questions got worse and the support became less day by day. Mike left us one year after his terminal diagnosis and I had to take two weeks off to try to get my head around my soulmate no longer being here. I was emotionally drained and mentally only able to concentrate for a few hours, and each day was different. I was asked to go to the boardroom with my managers one day. They said, "You are making people in the office uncomfortable. We thought you would be back to normal by now – you knew this was coming."

'After the way they reacted to Mike's death and the lack of support they gave me, it was not an environment I could stay in. I left the corporate work environment and created a start-up, founding MyMuse, which educates and trains organisations and senior management on how to support and navigate an employee being diagnosed with cancer or being a carer of someone with cancer.'

What helped

'I decided that Mike's death would be the inspiration to do something that helped others. Knowing his legacy would live on has kept me going. It's not always possible to quit without another job lined up, but if you are struggling with grief in an unsupportive work environment, it's okay to prioritise your mental health and give yourself some time to reassess what you need.'

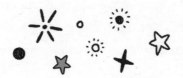

WHEN YOU'RE NOT COPING WELL AT WORK

People might assume that grief only lasts a few months or so, but, as we know, that's not the case. Grief is always with you. Although it evolves and can become somewhat easier to manage, for many, it can still feel difficult even years after the loss. If you've been back at work for a while but are still finding it hard to cope, it's important to seek support. The following tips might help.

- **Don't be afraid to ask for help.** Speak to your HR department or manager to see if they can arrange bereavement counselling sessions for you. Alternatively, you might like to organise to speak to a professional outside of work. Either way, talking to an expert who can give you tools and strategies to cope is an important step.

- **Be honest.** Let your employer know that you're struggling and give examples. If there are certain tasks that you're finding hard, let them know. Or, if it's the social side of work – whether that's putting on a brave face or dealing with prying colleagues – they might be able to help create some solutions to make your days a little easier.

- **Confide in your family and friends.** If you're finding work a challenge, it can help to share what's going on for you with those closest to you. Not only does it feel good to express your feelings, but they might be able to offer advice or, at the very least, a warm hug.

- **Plan things to look forward to.** This might be as simple as getting a take-away coffee in the morning, going to your favourite cafe for lunch, seeing a friend after work, or booking time off. Having some things to look forward to at the end of the working day, or in the future, can make things a little easier to bear.

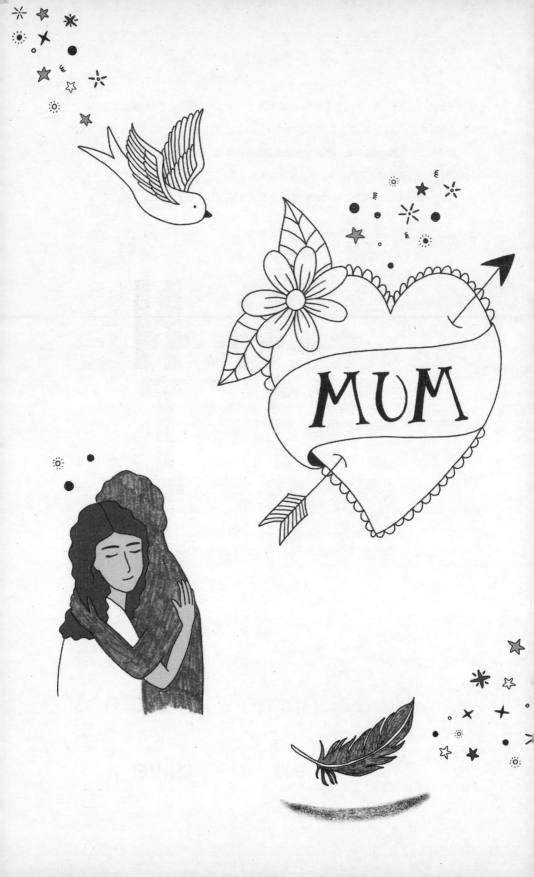

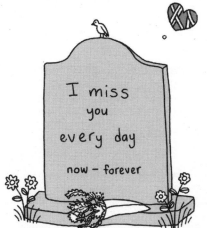

8.
GONE, BUT NOT FORGOT-TEN

Managing milestones and keeping memories alive

WHEN SOMEONE YOU LOVE DIES, IT CAN BE HARD TO WRAP YOUR HEAD AROUND THE FACT THAT THEY'RE GONE.

The thought of never seeing them, hearing their voice, or feeling their touch again can feel frightening. As we continue to learn to live our lives around our loss, we never stop missing them. And while throughout this book we've talked about different ways to cope with grief, there's an element of loss that's important to embrace, not overcome: the memory of our loved ones.

As we mentioned in Chapter 1, there's an assumption that to heal or cope with loss, you must find a point of closure to be able to move on with your life. There will always be moments that we want to share with the people who are no longer here. And in those moments, there will always be a tinge of sadness. The thought of moving on can feel distressing because grief often serves as a reminder that they were real. Why would we want to let that go? It might bring you comfort to know that you don't have to ever move on or let go. If anything, there should be less forgetting and more connecting. Keeping them alive in our hearts and minds is a fundamental part of living with loss.

For both of us, the way we've discovered a little bit of 'good' in our mourning is by finding ways to continue to express our love for our mums and include them in our lives through rituals and connecting with them via signs. Both our mums loved op-shopping, so we go op-shopping in their honour and feel close to them when we do. We listen to music that they loved and watch their favourite TV shows. We write to them and talk about them at every opportunity. We don't just do this on anniversaries or milestones, but every day. As we'll explore, there are loads of simple ways that you can honour your loved ones and embrace their memory, too.

Life without your person may very well feel like it sucks right now, and there is a brutal finality to death that can feel almost impossible to comprehend. But we promise you this: the relationship doesn't end after the funeral. And while there's no way out or over your loss, there is a way forwards without leaving your loved one behind.

'DEATHIVERSARIES' AND OTHER MILESTONE DAYS

Motherf*cking milestone days. Let's be real – every day, week or month after they died seems like a milestone, doesn't it? Looking at the calendar and realising how long it's been since you last heard their voice, or felt their touch, can be a significant shock as time goes by. Not having your person there to witness both the big and small life moments is painful.

There are lots of days that can be a trigger for grief – the date that they died, anniversaries, their birthday, *your* birthday, Mother's Day, Father's Day, family celebrations, holidays, weddings – the list goes on. Significant days can evoke strong emotions and grief bombs can strike hard around these times. We have both found that the lead-up to a milestone day can be harder than the day itself. The weeks prior can feel super griefy and like a cascade of emotions could spill out at any time. During these times, the reminders also feel constant (maybe because it's all we can think about). We know it's coming, so we're on edge and full of anticipation. One thing that can help in the lead-up is taking away any added pressure to feel like you have to 'nail' it or do something grand. Go easy on yourself and roll with how you feel on the day. Don't put pressure on yourself to come out all guns blazing with honouring them if you don't feel up to it. It's okay to sit out the occasion if it feels too hard to acknowledge. You're allowed to do that.

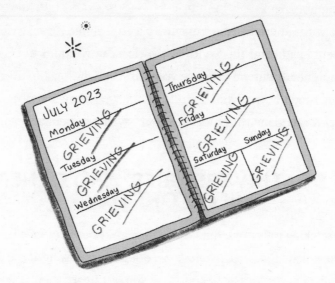

Above all, it's important to take care of yourself and do what you need. Do you want to stay in bed and forget that it's the day they died? Perfectly okay. Prefer to do nothing but scream into a pillow? Go for it. Would you rather crack on with work and pretend like everything's fine? Fair enough. Whatever you need to do for yourself to survive the day, do it! You get to write the rules when it comes to the way you honour your person and how you spend your time.

If you do want to mark a milestone, trying to work out what to do can be overwhelming. So, with the help of our community, here are some ideas that might inspire you.

- Talk about them (until the cows come home!).
- Buy yourself a bunch of their favourite flowers and put them in a fancy vase.
- Buy yourself a nice candle and light it for them.
- Cook their favourite meal or buy the snacks they loved. You could host a dinner party in their memory, or enjoy it solo.
- Listen to their favourite music (and if the tears start flowing, don't hold them back).
- Bake their favourite cake if it's their birthday. You could even sing 'Happy Birthday' (if it feels right).
- Heck, why not get a tattoo in their honour? Im got her mum's handwriting, and Sal got a tattoo of a rose (her mum's name).
- Create a memory box. You could include photos, cards, letters or little things that remind you of them.
- Let yourself *feel* the emotions and have a 'grief sesh' (for a refresher on this, skip back to page 69).
- Get together with family and friends and swap stories.
- Put on your PJs, get cosy and have a movie marathon, watching their favourite films.
- Talk to them out loud – don't be afraid to have a natter and let them know how you're feeling.
- Write about them, or to them. Take the time to reflect and express your feelings.
- Channel them by spending time doing something they loved.
- Visit their grave or the spot where their ashes are scattered. Cry, scream, reflect, shout . . . all at the same time, if you feel like it.

Ellie's experience with milestones

'My dad died suddenly when I was 14 years old and milestones have always been difficult for me, as they often bring back that physical pain of grief. More recently, I marked a big and scary-sounding milestone of the ten-year anniversary of Dad's death. This was particularly anxiety-inducing for me and in the lead-up I was doing a lot of thinking as to how I could best cope with the apprehension, fear and frustration that is associated with the anniversary of that dreaded day.

'I have found that there's often a lot of pressure placed on these milestones: pressure to mark the day with some sort of grand gesture, or pressure to feel a certain way, whether that's happy and joyful for the life that you shared, or angry and griefy.'

What helped

'On the most recent milestone, instead of feeling pressure to be a certain way, I broke it down into chunks over a couple of days. I did things that would make me feel closer to my dad, including listening to his favourite music and saying a few words to him, in the hope that he'd be listening.'

GRIEF TIP — Give yourself permission to be a hot mess! Lower your expectations of yourself around milestone days. Things that you are normally able to do might feel hard or even impossible. That's okay.

Surviving the holidays ('tis the season to feel griefy!)

As well as milestone days, the holiday season can be a time of year when it feels like an onslaught of grief. Christmas, in particular, might feel less like 'ho-ho-ho' and more like 'no-no-no'. It's a time of year when memories can hit us hard, and we're constantly reminded that our person isn't here to celebrate with us. You might feel pressured to be festive when all you want to do is hide from the world. Remember how we talked about self-care and setting boundaries in Chapter 4? It's important at this time of year to practise both, so you don't get completely overwhelmed.

Here are some ways to look after yourself during holiday seasons.

COMMUNICATE WHAT YOU NEED TO OTHERS

If your capacity for festive activities is low, don't be afraid to let people you trust know, so they can support you. Try saying, 'Do you know what? I'm not feeling festive this year. I want to keep things low-key, but I would still like your support. Maybe we can do quieter, slower-paced things.' Being open can take the pressure off feeling like you have to put on a brave face and fake any festive cheer.

WORK TOGETHER – AS A FAMILY, AS FRIENDS OR AS PARTNERS

Decide whether you're going to do anything to remember your loved one. Don't leave it unsaid before the day itself. Emotions can be heightened during the festive season and misunderstandings can happen. So, if you want to do something, get it out in the open. Have a chat and be upfront and that way everyone feels included.

DON'T OVERCOMMIT

If you know that, deep down, you don't have the energy, be honest. Instead of packing your schedule full, let others know that you only have the headspace to spend a few hours together, or that you can't attend every gathering or social event. Flag that you might need to leave early, or cancel at the last minute.

SAY NO

If the thought of socialising brings you out in a cold sweat, it's a good idea to put some boundaries in place. Prioritise yourself and your energy levels. It's okay to politely decline invitations, or say no to having guests over if it will drain your battery. Also, if certain people make you feel uncomfortable, put a limit on how often you see them (if at all).

Talking of carrying traditions forwards, although our mums were both very untraditional when it came to the holiday season, we still incorporate their unusual (but cute) untraditions. Im's mum, Vanessa, never had a Christmas tree, but each year used to decorate a big twig with tinsel and baubles. She thought it was 'arty'. Sal's mum, Rose, also bucked the trend with her Christmas tree, putting a stuffed Miss Piggy toy on top instead of an angel. Our mums often couldn't be bothered to cook a Christmas dinner – maybe it's because neither of them had an oven (another random thing they had in common!). So, over in the UK, Sal's mum would sometimes make a turkey curry. In Australia, Im's mum would make salads and they'd eat them around a coffee table, sitting on the floor. We miss their anti-Christmas traditions as much as we miss them, and now we carry them forwards – twig, pig and all.

New Year grief

Christmas is followed up straight away by another marker in the calendar that can feel unpredictably griefy – New Year. Great, huh?! You got yourself to the other side of Christmas and you're thinking, *I've survived. I'm through the worst of it*. And then, almost straight away, 31 December hits. It can feel like a big reminder that you're facing another year without your person. It's a new year, but it's the same old grief.

Looking into the year ahead without your person can feel overwhelming. You may still be feeling very raw and the thought of people celebrating *anything* right now feels completely wrong. Fireworks – what for? Your world feels like it's over. Stupid little party hats and sparklers – why? You literally can't even think about the next minute, let alone a whole year without them! Just remember, as much as it may feel like it, moving into a new year does not mean you're leaving them behind.

As time ticks on and your grief remains, it can feel like you are moving further and further away from your loved one and the memories you hold close. You may have spent the countdown scream-crying into your wine glass, or maybe you went to bed early to try to avoid it all, only to wake up the next morning to all the 'Happy New Year' and 'New Year, New Me' posts plastered over social media. People around you may be comparing New Year's resolutions (that they likely never follow through with anyway), but all you are trying to do is survive.

Coming from two grievers, the absolute last thing we felt like doing on New Year's Day was setting resolutions, or revamping our to-do lists. We're not really into resolutions, but here are some small (and realistic) goals that you might want to try, to help you cope with your grief as you roll into a new year.

- Focus on taking each day as it comes.
- Start prioritising yourself and *your* needs.

- Incorporate a small self-care 'micro-ritual' into your day (see page 143).
- Journal twice a week to help process your emotions.
- Move your body for 30 minutes a day.
- Limit screen time 30 minutes before bed to get a better night's sleep.
- Ask for help if you feel overwhelmed, or take three things off your weekly to-do list.
- Limit caffeine and booze if they make you feel crap.
- Let go of any unrealistic expectations you have put on yourself.
- Try to set boundaries where you need to (and stick to them).

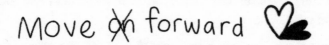

Move ~~on~~ forward 💙

IF

all you

did today

WAS PUT
ON PANTS,
YOU'RE
DOING AN

amazing job!

What our community said about . . .

CREATING NEW HOLIDAY TRADITIONS

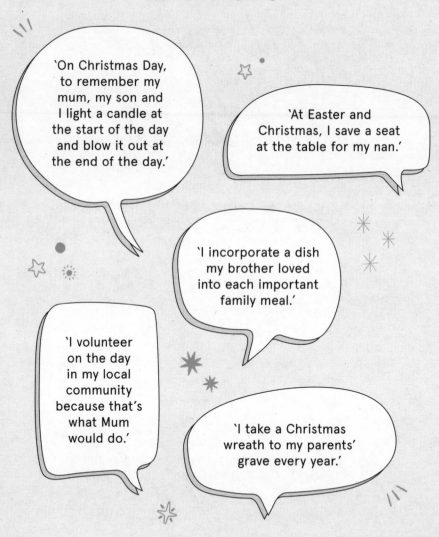

'On Christmas Day, to remember my mum, my son and I light a candle at the start of the day and blow it out at the end of the day.'

'At Easter and Christmas, I save a seat at the table for my nan.'

'I incorporate a dish my brother loved into each important family meal.'

'I volunteer on the day in my local community because that's what Mum would do.'

'I take a Christmas wreath to my parents' grave every year.'

'I give a toast to my husband each year. He always did the toast at Christmas dinner. Now, it's an important part of keeping him included in the day.'

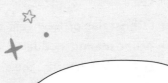

'I rally the troops and we spend the day together in the lead-up to Christmas. We have a festival in honour of our friend, share memories, listen to music and drink wine. It helps us all feel close to each other, and to her.'

'Every year, I buy my daughter presents she would love and put them under the tree.'

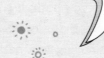

'Even though it's been years, I always write a Christmas card to my sister and take it to her resting place. If I feel up to it, I read it out loud.'

COPING DURING OTHER TOUGH HOLIDAYS

It's not just Christmas or New Year's that can bring up grief. There are other loaded holidays, such as Valentine's Day, Mother's Day and Father's Day, too. Some ways that you might like to support yourself on these days include:

GATHER A CREW
Maybe you have friends who have lost someone, who also find certain holidays hard. Host a gathering and indulge in something nice together, or at the very least, spend the day supporting each other.

ORGANISE A DAY IN THEIR HONOUR
Plan a day doing the things your person loved, or things that meant something to you both. If you have kids or grandkids, you might like to get them involved with the planning, too. Spend the day channelling your person and celebrating them.

VOLUNTEER
Helping others can give you a sense of purpose on days you might want to forget. Find a cause that matters to you, or that mattered to your person, and see if you can spend the day doing good for others.

TREAT IT LIKE A NORMAL DAY
Hallmark holidays are hard, and you might find that you want to forget they are even happening. It's okay to ignore them!

CONTINUING THE BOND WITH EVERYDAY RITUALS

Connecting with your loved one doesn't have to be something you only do on milestone days or during the holiday season. You don't have to *only* honour them on days that feel big. You can find little ways to make them part of your everyday life, too. This can be especially helpful if you're struggling with the difficult feelings of finality after loss, as it can help you to feel like they are still included in your life.

There's a concept that we've found super helpful in reframing how we keep our mums part of our everyday lives. It's called the 'continuing bonds' theory, and it was explained by Klass, Silverman and Nickman in their 1996 book, *Continuing Bonds: New understandings of grief*. The crux of the concept is that just because our loved ones aren't here physically anymore, it doesn't mean that they didn't exist (and it sure as hell doesn't mean we need to 'let go' of them to be grieving successfully). The authors suggest that you can still create a bond with the person who died and that it's a healthy way to grieve. Healthy grief, they say, is not resolved by detaching from the deceased, but instead by creating a new relationship with those who are no longer with us.

We both *love* this theory because, ultimately, it's about readjusting to life as it is now and finding new ways to reimagine the relationship you have with your person. It's not weird or unhealthy to continue the relationship with them – it's an important part of grief. We both create moments in our weeks, even when life gets busy, to continue the bond with our mums.

Sal

I brought some of my mum's ashes back to Australia with me and scattered them at a beautiful headland overlooking a beach close to where I live. I've made it a weekly ritual to walk 30 minutes along the beach and up to the headland to the spot where they are scattered to say hello. Sometimes I'll sit and talk to my mum, sometimes I'll reflect and remember, and sometimes – on the extra-griefy days – I cry. Even though she's not physically here, having a special spot where I can connect to her makes me feel like she's close by.

Im

Keeping my mum connected to my daughter is super important to me. I always talk about Mum and say things like, 'Your grandma would love that' or, if we saw a butterfly I would say, 'There's Grandma coming to say hello.' One night, my daughter picked up a bit of sock lint and shouted, 'Mum! It's Grandma coming to see me!' She was so excited. Although it's (hilariously) heartbreaking, I find those moments beautiful as I like to believe my daughter can feel my mum's energy around her.

You don't have to feel pressure to create purpose from your pain. You don't need to transform your grief into something. It's okay to just *grieve*.

Simple rituals

There are some easy ways that you can incorporate rituals into your day-to-day life to feel connected to your person.

TALK TO THEM

Have a chat with them out loud or in your head. Tell them what's going on for you. Share your news, tell them about your day or new ways you're coping with your grief. It can bring comfort and make them feel close.

ASK THEM FOR ADVICE

Next time you have a decision to make, include them in it. Think about what advice they would give. What would their take on the situation be? What would they say? It can make you feel that they are close and ease the decision-making process a little.

WEAR SOMETHING OF THEIRS

Putting on a piece of jewellery, an accessory or an item of clothing that was theirs can feel like they are close and connected to you, because it's a part of them that you can touch and feel.

TAKE ON A HOBBY THAT THEY ENJOYED

Some of our podcast listeners have taken up the hobbies of their loved ones, including football, piano lessons and Pilates. Learning something they enjoyed might teach you a few new things about them and can be a way to feel that you are carrying their passions forwards.

VOLUNTEER FOR A CAUSE THEY CARED ABOUT

This could be once a month or perhaps just on, or around, milestone days. You could also make donations to a charity that was close to their heart.

What our community said about...

CREATING EVERYDAY RITUALS

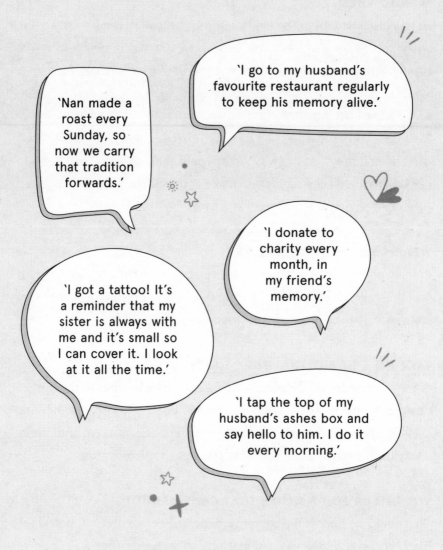

'I go to my husband's favourite restaurant regularly to keep his memory alive.'

'Nan made a roast every Sunday, so now we carry that tradition forwards.'

'I donate to charity every month, in my friend's memory.'

'I got a tattoo! It's a reminder that my sister is always with me and it's small so I can cover it. I look at it all the time.'

'I tap the top of my husband's ashes box and say hello to him. I do it every morning.'

'To feel close to my friend, I crack open a bottle of wine, put on her favourite music and cook one of her legendary recipes.'

'I've made my mum's favourite perfume my scent. Smell is the strongest of the sense memories, so I wear it every day and it makes me feel closer to her.'

'When we were growing up, Grandad used to buy us doughnuts for breakfast every weekend. So now we do it!'

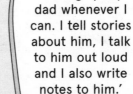

'I bring up my dad whenever I can. I tell stories about him, I talk to him out loud and I also write notes to him.'

'Each morning, I say three things about my mum that I was grateful for.'

Psychologist Tamara's view on maintaining a connection

Thankfully, grief support has come a long way. Long-held views about grief have been rejected, with research failing to support popular notions that grief is a predictable and staged emotional journey from distress to 'recovery'. It is only in recent decades that we've shifted from the concept that successful grieving requires someone to formally 'let go' of their attachment and connection to the deceased and 'move on', to the concept that while death ends a life, it does not necessarily end a relationship and that this can be beneficial for those still living.

The development of a continued bond can be conscious and can be expressed in many different ways. Studies have found that approximately half of people going through bereavement experience the sense of presence of the deceased. You may experience the deceased by visiting their grave, in your dreams, feeling their presence or through participating in religious or spiritual rituals or linking objects to them.

Research shows that spontaneous and facilitated after-death communication is beneficial. Some ways of doing this include writing letters to your loved one, sharing stories about them with others or speaking to them directly or to photos. A more subtle way can be practising values they embodied, such as doing a charitable deed or making a conscious effort with another person. Many people build the connection through significant life milestones, such as birthdays, weddings and anniversaries, or by wearing something that reminds them of their loved one.

BE THE THINGS YOU *loved most* ABOUT THE PEOPLE WHO ARE GONE.

– UNKNOWN

Madelaine's experience with rituals

'In March 2021, my beautiful husband Ricky went to work and never came home. He was involved in an accident in his work truck on the way to a job and passed away instantly, leaving behind myself and our then five-month-old daughter, Sienna. My entire world came crashing down. I remember thinking, *What now?* Ricky was my best friend, my protector, my safe place and my soulmate, and had been for nine years. He's the first man Sienna ever loved – how do I tell her that her daddy is just gone?

'I decided I had to make a choice. I could allow the negative thoughts to consume me, or I could channel my pain into living and breathing for Ricky. My purpose now is to live in honour of him, so Sienna knows how special her father truly was.'

What helped

'I have several rituals to ensure Ricky remains present in our everyday lives. We talk about him and share memories that make everyone smile. We set him a place at the dinner table with his photo and favourite beer. We kiss his picture and tell him we love him every day. It's extremely important to me that Sienna knows he's still the most important man in her life and that he loves her unconditionally.'

What are the top three things you loved most about your person, that you can carry forwards?

DOING DEATH DIFFERENTLY

We've already talked about how the Western world seeks to limit expressions of grief. Other cultures can have very different ways of dealing with loss. Their mourning rituals may help you rethink how to remember your loved one.

In Māori culture, the dead play an important role in traditions. The tangihanga (often called tangi for short), is the traditional Māori ceremony to mourn someone who has died. The deceased lie in an open casket, often in the wharenui (a large, communal house) and family members lie beside the casket to weep and sing. Other members of the community will also sleep in the wharenui along with the dead body. And, at all gatherings and meetings, no matter the nature, the dead are acknowledged through whaikōrero (speeches), karanga (calls), songs and tears. Remembering those who have passed reminds the living of the importance of life, relationships and community.

Community is an important part of Indigenous Australian traditions around death, too. 'Sorry business' is the term that refers to funerals and mourning the death of a community member, and while rituals and practices may be unique to each area, funerals and mourning are a communal activity and can last days (or sometimes even weeks).

Mexican culture celebrates the annual 'Day of the Dead' to honour their ancestors. People set up an altar with candles so the spirits can find their way home. Some include items that were important to their loved ones when they were alive, or the favourite food of the deceased. They also have a party at the gravesite and create life-sized papier-mâché skeletons, which serve as a reminder that death is very much a part of life, and not something to be feared.

Jewish tradition has 'shiva', which is a week-long mourning period that commences at home after the burial. It is a time for family members to embrace and comfort each other and discuss the loss. It's a way to remember the person who died, and express sorrow.

HELLO FROM THE OTHER SIDE

It wouldn't be a chapter on keeping a connection without talking about two of our favourite topics: the afterlife and asking for signs. Connecting through signs from the 'other side' is something that has brought both of us, and many of our listeners, a bit of comfort in our grief, and it's one of the most requested topics on the podcast. One of the main reasons that many of us take solace in signs is that they bring hope that our person is still around us. It's special to think we can still have a relationship with them.

Not everyone believes in the afterlife or signs, and that's okay. As we mentioned at the start of this book, it's a bit of a 'choose your own adventure' when it comes to the way we do this whole grief thing. What works for some, may not work for others. So, if signs aren't your jam, we respect that. However, if you read on with a bit of an open mind, you may at the very least find it intriguing to learn about the experiences of others.

Have you watched the Netflix documentary, *Surviving Death*? We interviewed award-winning journalist Leslie Kean, author of the fascinating book, *Surviving Death: A journalist investigates evidence for an afterlife*, which was the inspiration behind the documentary. We spoke in depth about signs, mediumship, near-death experiences and reincarnation, and it's safe to say we were both blown away. What makes Leslie's work so fascinating is that when she started writing her book, she was a sceptic. Being an investigative journalist, her work is grounded in evidence-based research and hard facts. Yet, when interviewing leading doctors, psychiatrists and academics, Leslie experienced things that shifted her perspective on whether consciousness survives death. Asking for signs, and receiving them, was one of them – even though they aren't strictly evidential, they were so personal and specific to her, which brought her a lot of comfort in her grief.

During our fascinating conversation, Leslie shared how, by communicating through signs, she has strengthened her relationship with her brother who died. Leslie had a reading with world-renowned psychic medium and author of the must-read book, *Signs: The secret language of the universe*, Laura Lynne Jackson, who told her that the sign to look out for when her brother was trying to communicate with her was a red balloon. About a week later, Leslie was meditating in the evening and asked her brother to please send her a physical sign so that she knew it was all real. When Leslie woke up the next morning, she looked outside and there was a bunch of red balloons caught in the tree, right outside her window. Leslie said she feels like she has a new relationship with her brother now, and in some ways, it's more profound than it was when he was alive.

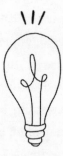

Connecting with our loved ones via signs

Like Leslie, communicating with our mums through signs has been a big part of feeling connected with them. When we interviewed Laura Lynne Jackson for our podcast, she explained that our loved ones are working hard to create this new language with us through signs, to help us understand that they are still with us.

Laura explained that signs are a method of communication from the other side, like a secret language we can co-create. Opening your heart and mind to the language of signs can help strengthen the connection with your loved one on the other side and, as Leslie experienced, it can create a new relationship with them. The force behind signs, Laura explained, is energy.

At first, 'default signs' are often sent to us. They are easier for us to recognise and for our loved one to put in our path. Not every sign needs to be what Laura calls a 'showstopper' – they can be subtle things you might otherwise miss but that can have meaning, such as coins appearing in our path, a sequence of numbers, slogans, licence plates, music, butterflies, feathers or electrical disturbances. Then there are what Laura calls 'distinct signs', which are the specific signs we request, however unusual or obscure – perhaps a word, an object, a movie or a song.

Sometimes these signs might appear at significant times, such as a birthday or anniversary. The other side is always trying to communicate with us, according to Laura, so it's important to be receptive and pay attention.

There are no rules on what a sign should look like, but if you're asking for one, it should be something specific, such as their favourite flower, an inside joke or a cartoon. Laura recommends crafting a message clear enough that you know it when you see it. This will increase the feelings of love and connection that come when you do receive it. You can just say, 'I really need you to send me [insert specific thing].' The golden rules, she says, are to be clear, be specific and be patient. There's no limit to the number of signs you can ask for and it doesn't always have to be the same thing. The more signs you ask for, according to Laura, the bigger the language you co-create.

A common question we hear from our listeners when we cover this topic is, 'What if I ask for a sign and I don't get it?' We asked Laura why some people might not get their sign and she said it's easy to miss them. A lot of times our loved ones will send them in very creative ways. Laura shared a story about her mum asking for a purple elephant from her dad who had died. One afternoon, Laura's sister realised that her mum had driven straight past a restaurant called The Purple Elephant, which had a huge purple elephant statue out the front. Her mum completely missed it. The lesson: you need not just to look, but to see. To do this, you don't need to change anything about your life except to slightly alter your method of perception.

In her book, *Signs*, Laura says that in the sport of golf, positive-thinking coaches tell golfers to walk down the fairway with their heads held high, fully absorbing the landscape around them. This is designed to get them more involved and alert and receptive, and better prepared for their next shot. She explains that we can do the same in our everyday lives – we can fully absorb the landscape around us by simply looking up, which can make you better prepared for the sign when it comes.

If you are asking for signs from your loved one and feeling frustrated because you are not getting them, here are a few things Laura suggests you try:

BE DIRECT AND CLEAR

When communicating with the other side about how you'd like to receive your sign, say to them, in your thoughts, *I know you are probably sending signs, but I am missing them. Can you please deliver my sign through someone saying it verbally to me?*

UNDERSTAND THAT IT'S A CO-CREATIVE LANGUAGE

Your loved one might choose a sign of their own that they are known for. For example, if they loved a certain song, they might send you that song. Or, if they loved the colour pink, you might see pink everywhere that day. If they had a nickname for you, you might hear it somewhere.

MAKE IT DISTINCT

Laura suggests the more creative or outlandish the signs we ask for, the better. The more unusual and unique to you, the better the chance you have of spotting it.

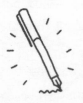

What sign could you ask for? What's something that's unique to you and your person? Write it down, then ask for it aloud. Remember: be clear, be specific and be patient.

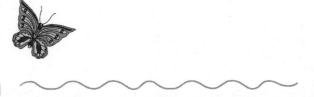

Im

Around eight months after Mum died, we held a memorial for her at one of her best friend's properties. We planted a flame tree in her honour. It was a beautiful, yet sad day.

My mum's name is Vanessa, which is of Greek origin, and the meaning of Vanessa is 'butterfly'. Even when she was alive, she would tell me that she was a butterfly and I was a dragonfly, so they are both very symbolic to me. We all wore butterfly clips on the day, and as we arrived at the spot where we were about to plant the tree, hundreds of white butterflies appeared out of nowhere and were swirling around us all. It was pure magic. I'll never forget it. We all stopped in our tracks and looked at each other, knowing with absolute certainty that it was her. She was there and it gave me so much comfort in the moment. Even for a split-second, feeling like she was around me in some form was such a gift.

Sal

My mum's nickname when she was growing up was Mouse. One day, I was driving to Im's to record a podcast interview. I was feeling particularly griefy and so, out loud, I asked my mum to send me a sign to show me she was around. I asked for a mouse. An hour later, I arrived at Im's and the first thing I saw was one of her daughter's toys on the living room floor – a stuffed toy mouse. I smiled at the thought that it was a nod from Mum, letting me know she was close.

Helen's experience with signs

'I was somebody who fell into the "sceptic" category when it came to my beliefs about the possibility of receiving signs from passed loved ones. It was a couple of months since my dad had died and the world was still in lockdown. My fiancé Leigh had gone into a pharmacy for me while I waited on a bench outside. I was overcome with emotion, trying not to be the girl crying in public. I looked up to the sky. "Pops, please send me a sign. Send me a white feather to let me know you're here, but it can't just be a random one on the street. I need it to be sent to me so clearly that I know for a fact it's 100 per cent you."

'We'd left the patio door open that connects to the lounge room. When we returned home and stepped into the room, it happened: a white feather flew in through the tiny gap of the patio door, swirled around the air and landed smack bang in the middle of the floor. I couldn't believe it! Whenever I doubt the possibility of life after death, I remember this experience and numerous similar ones that have followed. My belief now is that if something brings you comfort and feels like it could be a sign from your loved one, then a sign it is, no doubt or explanation needed.'

Ebony's experience with signs

'I lost my big brother, Christian, in January 2022 after a six-month illness – he was only 44. He was also only weeks away from being eligible for an organ transplant, and his medical team was looking at fast-tracking the process if he pulled through. He was courageous until the end and although it was the hardest experience, I am grateful I was by his side at the hospital as he took his last breath.

'My brother took a lot of pride in his sexuality – he loved the rainbow flag and all that it represented. As soon as we got in the car to drive home from the hospital that evening, "Over the Rainbow" came on the radio. My partner commented that it was such a strange song to be playing and that he'd never heard it on the radio before. The next day, we received flowers with a beautiful card that said, "He'll be with us somewhere over the rainbow." When Christian first got sick and the prognosis was looking grim, he had given a friend the list of music that he wanted to be played at his memorial. The following day we received the song list and, sure enough, "Over the Rainbow" was on it.

'After Christian's memorial service, we were sitting at my parents' house when my partner was drawn to go outside and look up – of course, a beautiful rainbow was in the sky. In the days that followed they appeared frequently – I've never seen so many rainbows as I have since Christian passed away.

'The rainbow quickly became a clear, strong sign from Christian, so I decided to get a small rainbow tattoo on my wrist. It brings me comfort and feels like I have something from him with me always.'

CONCLUSION
Grieving with love

You did it – you made it to the end of the book. Although, this isn't the end at all. In many ways, it's the beginning – the start of your new relationship with the elephant in the room (aka your grief).

You've likely heard the phrase, 'Time heals all wounds'. Frankly, we think that's BS. Time does not diminish grief. It will always be there, ebbing and flowing as we live our lives. Grief isn't a task that you tick off your to-do list or something that you have to get over. It's a life-long process of adjustment and integration, and that's okay.

Maybe in time, we grieve less with pain and more with love. This concept was shared with us by David Kessler when we asked him about the timelines people put on grief and grieving. He explained that when people ask him how long they are going to grieve for, he asks them: 'How long is a person going to be dead? If they've been dead for a long time, then you will grieve for a long time. It doesn't mean you will always grieve with pain. You may in time grieve with love.' For us, that's the ultimate goal in grief.

In author Nora McInerny's viral TED talk, 'We don't "move on" from grief. We move forwards with it', she explains that some things can't be fixed, and not all wounds are meant to heal. She describes grief as a 'multitasking emotion', and says that 'you can and will be sad and happy; you'll be grieving, and able to love in the same year or week, the same breath. We need to remember that a grieving person is going to laugh again and smile again. If they're lucky, they'll even find love again . . . yes, absolutely, they're going to move forwards. But that doesn't mean that they've moved on.' Mic drop, Nora!

As you learn to move forwards with your grief, eventually you may just find a little bit of 'good' in your mourning. It might be a new perspective, a glimmer of hope, or even a moment of joy. And while the pain may soften over time, grief doesn't disappear. It is, in essence, an expression of our love. So, in many ways, why would we want it to disappear?

We hope that reading this book has given you the encouragement that you can survive this. Maybe it's given you a fresh outlook, or even a little laugh at times. Grief is undoubtedly one of the toughest life-changing experiences we will all face, yet here you are, despite it all. And going forwards, do us a favour and give yourself a little more self-compassion, because you deserve it.

Showing up every day after a loss takes courage. Reading this book takes courage. Embracing grief in all its unpredictability takes courage. When it comes to healing, it's easy to get so caught up in how much further there is to go that you lose sight of how far you've already come. Be proud of yourself.

On days when you're feeling in the thick of your grief and like no-one understands, flick through these pages, because we do understand. Come back to us when you need some solidarity and a reminder that you are not alone. As you continue this journey, remember that we're standing on the sidelines cheering for you.

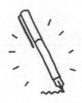

Take some time to think about your grief and what it means to you. In a month, come back to your journal and ask yourself this same question, and notice any shifts in your thoughts and feelings.

What our community said about . . .

GRIEVING WITH LOVE

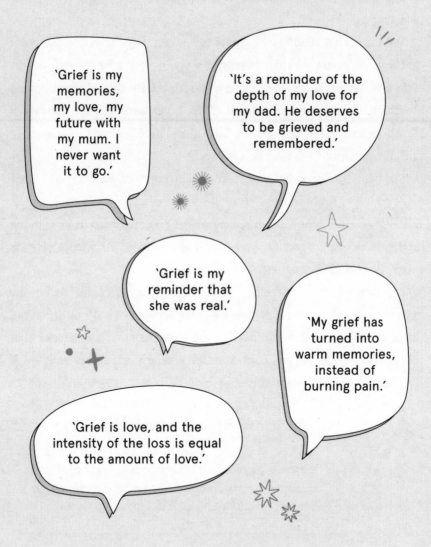

'Grief is my memories, my love, my future with my mum. I never want it to go.'

'It's a reminder of the depth of my love for my dad. He deserves to be grieved and remembered.'

'Grief is my reminder that she was real.'

'My grief has turned into warm memories, instead of burning pain.'

'Grief is love, and the intensity of the loss is equal to the amount of love.'

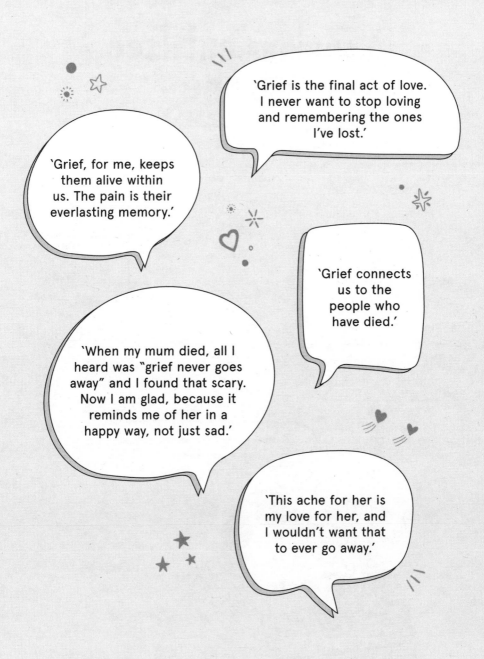

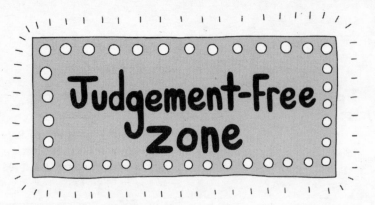

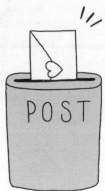

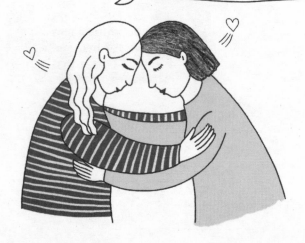

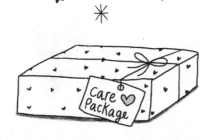

TIPS FOR YOUR SUPPORT TEAM

Advice for your partner, family, friends or colleagues

HEY, SUPPORTER. IF YOU'RE HELPING
SOMEONE YOU CARE ABOUT COPE
WITH LOSS, OR MAYBE YOU WANT
TO LEARN MORE ABOUT GRIEF,
THANK YOU FOR READING THIS.

Let's start by being real. It can be hard to know what to do or say when faced with death. None of it is easy, for anyone involved. And when it comes to supporting someone in grief, it can feel unbearable to witness others in intense pain. You might feel helpless, awkward or be worried you'll say something that doesn't land quite as intended. It scares you off, so you don't do or say anything. Easier that way, right?

Wrong.

You don't need to be perfect or know all the right things to say or do. You don't have to fly in like a superhero and fix everything because you can't. You don't need to make the pain go away, because it won't. But don't worry, there are things that you can do in a loving and awesome way to ease teeny moments of pain for the person grieving. Grief isn't something that goes away. It lasts a lifetime. While over time the intensity of the heartache and pain might get easier to carry, grief is always there, in the background. There's no 'one size fits all' to grief support, and that is a-okay. Allow us to share a collection of our favourite ways to give someone who's grieving the extra care they need.

REAL TALK IS WELCOME

Talking about death – and grief – is hard. On top of knowing whether it's the right time to reach out, it can be hard to know what to say when someone dies. You might feel pressure to reel off something profound or use flowery language. No need! Be straightforward and honest. Acknowledge that you feel awkward. For example, you could say, 'I'm rubbish at knowing the right thing to say in these situations, but I want you to know I am sorry.' Just be real – no need to sugarcoat it.

IN THE WEEK AFTER THE DEATH

REACH OUT

If you live with the person or see them a lot, or if the loss isn't recent, then skip this part.

One of the best things you can do to support someone in the early days is simply to reach out and acknowledge what they are going through. Don't stay silent! Call them, send a text or write a card or note. If you're hesitant about whether it's the right time, know that it's never too soon to let them know you are thinking of them. Don't let feeling a little uncomfortable stop you from getting in touch. Showing the person that you acknowledge and accept their loss can mean a lot.

SEND A SYMPATHY CARD

Don't underestimate the power of a sympathy card. Cards can bring so much comfort and be an incredible source of strength to the person who is grieving. If you feel a bit awkward about putting pen to paper, don't worry. The key is to focus on the person you are writing to. Think, *What can I say that will offer some comfort?* You could share a fond memory of the person who died or keep it simple and let them know that you are there for them.

Instead of this   Say this

'I can't even imagine . . .' → 'This is shit. I know right now I can't make this better, but I have got your back through this, always.'

'My condolences to you and your family.' → 'There are no words for how hard this is. My thoughts are with you and your family and, when you need me, I am here.'

'So sorry for your loss.' → 'I am so sorry. None of this is fair. You are surrounded by love during this difficult time. I am just a phone call away. I will make myself available to you at any time.'

'My deepest sympathies.' → 'Things are really hard for you right now. I want you to know you are not alone, I am here for you, and I will help however I can.'

'It was their time to go.' → 'This absolutely sucks. I want you to know I am thinking of you every step of the way.'

TAKE A CARE PACKAGE

Sympathy card not your vibe? A thoughtful care package can be just as meaningful. Have a think about what the grieving person might like, or need, to make this tough time a teensy bit more comfortable.

Here are some ideas:

- a week's worth of home-cooked meals that they can easily freeze (the last thing a grieving person wants to do is cook – trust us!)
- some essential groceries – bread, milk, tea . . . and *lots* of chocolate
- they are probably going to feel exhausted, so a set of new pyjamas, a weighted blanket and an eye mask might help make sleep time a bit easier
- lavender oil, a fragrant candle and Epsom bath salts to help them relax
- if the situation is right, you could share some items from the person who died (belongings, photos or letters)
- a nice journal and pen for them to write down their thoughts and feelings.

 Be a point person. Something that can help is offering to communicate with others – for example, sharing updates and funeral details, so the griever doesn't have to worry about doing it.

OFFER PRACTICAL SUPPORT

After a death, there is so much to get done. There's endless admin and other things to sort out, such as cancelling accounts, organising the funeral and sorting belongings. On top of trying to process death and generally just survive, people might not have the capacity to think about even the smallest of chores.

As a supporter, one of the best things you can do is be proactive. Think about recurring tasks that they might need help with. But here's the most important part. Rather than saying, 'let me know what I can do' and then not following up, offer specific help and then take action. Don't just ask – *do*. Think about what you can take off their plate.

Here are some examples of helpful plate-clearers.

- 'I'd like to walk your dog for the next month. I can come over at 9 a.m. and 5 p.m. Is that okay?'
- 'Do you need any mail sending or picking up? I can swing by at 2 p.m. every Thursday.'
- 'Do you need your weekly shop doing? I can do this for you if you jot down a list. Or, I can have a look in your fridge and pantry.'
- 'I'd like to cook for you one night a week, for the next four weeks. What day works best for you?'

Don't just sweep in and take over without consent, no matter how well-meaning (unless you know the person really, really well). It's important to ask first.

ADD 'NO NEED TO REPLY'

After a death, people often receive loads of messages, voicemails and emails offering sympathy and kind words. Even though it's always really appreciated, it can feel overwhelming for the recipient to reply to them all. Make it easy for them by adding 'no need to reply' at the end of the message, so they know that any pressure to respond is off.

FOR ONGOING SUPPORT

DON'T TRY TO FIX IT

A lot of support and help can come in the form of telling people what they should do, or how they should feel. We know that you want to take away the pain. You might want to sweep in with a solution. Maybe you've got some suggestions on ways to cope that you think are helpful. As good as your intentions might be, if you're supporting someone, try not to tell them what they should be doing, or how they should be feeling. Sure, you might do things differently if you were in their shoes, but you're not. This is their loss.

TALK ABOUT THE PERSON WHO DIED

You might assume that grievers don't want to talk about the person who died. Not true! Talking about them is actually one of the best things you can do. It signals to the griever that you are keeping the memory of their person alive. Feel free to ask questions about their person and let them tell you all the stories. You could also share *your* favourite memory of them, too.

OFFER A JUDGEMENT-FREE ZONE

A really good way to support someone who is grieving is to be present, without judgement. Practise active listening with compassion and empathy, even if you don't *really* understand. Know that your presence is enough and listen without trying to find a reason. Put aside your desire to want to offer up solutions to fix anything – no reasoning, no questions, nothing. Honestly, it can truly transform the way you show up for someone experiencing loss.

If you are supporting someone, let them know that it's okay to feel sad and cry if they need to. Let them know they can come as they are and express how they feel.

SHOW UP . . . AND KEEP SHOWING UP

In the first few months after a loss, it's common for people to rally around a person. However, after the initial months, people tend to start dropping away as life resumes. Having a steadfast family member or friend to count on can really help. Be that person who keeps checking in. Be there when everyone else has moved on. Keep showing up, and do it for longer than you think is necessary.

And, if you choose to show up, be consistent! This one is a biggie – don't say you'll be there if you plan to cancel, because for the person going through loss, they might be looking forward to a much-needed break from their grief. Please, please, please don't flake on someone who is going through a loss.

KEEP ON COMMUNICATING

Grief is heavy and overwhelming, and it can vary in intensity from moment to moment. You might make a plan and then the person grieving cancels. You might text them and they don't reply. Don't take it personally, just remember that they have so much on their mind. One thing that you can do to be awesome support is to not give up (without being pushy, of course). Let them know it's fine if they cancel plans at the last minute, and that you'll still be there and will continue to invite them, even if they don't feel like it. Just keep reaching out, and longer than you think is necessary.

REPHRASE 'HOW ARE YOU?'

People might ask a griever, 'How are you?' or 'Are you okay?' Even though their heart probably feels so incredibly heavy, they might auto-respond with, 'Yeah, I'm fine, thanks.' Really, they are probably the furthest they can be from fine. 'Fine, thanks' could actually mean that things are bloody hard and they need help. It could mean that they are struggling to keep it together, but are scared to open up.

This is where you can step in and give them an opportunity to be honest. What can be really helpful is when people ask how you really are. Next time, try asking, 'How are you *today*?' By adding 'today', you are inviting the person to open up about how they are feeling in the moment. You signal that you are willing to actually hear how they are, giving them a cue that, if they want to, it's safe to open up. It can feel like a huge relief for a grieving person to have the opportunity to be honest about their emotions.

SUGGEST DOING QUIET THINGS

If you do meet up, understand that the person who is grieving might want to do something quiet. They might not want to talk about what is going on for them; if they do, it's best to suggest somewhere that is calm, like a quiet coffee shop or a park. You could suggest doing something that doesn't require a lot of talking, but where you can be present with them. Going to the cinema or theatre is a good idea, as it takes the pressure off talking, while also giving a welcome distraction or break.

AVOID PLATITUDES ('COS THEY HURT!)

Platitudes are phrases along the lines of, 'they're in a better place' or 'at least they are not in pain anymore'. They may seem like helpful things to say and come from a good place, but they can also make those who are struggling feel like their grief is being minimised or misunderstood, and can imply that their feelings aren't seen or heard. They might feel like they have to hide their pain, or pretend they are okay. You might be surprised to read this, as a lot of people don't realise the impacts these statements can have. But hey, it can be helpful to know the phrases that can really sting, right?

'At least' is one of the worst offenders when it comes to platitudes. For example, if you said 'at least you saw them before they died', it might come across as 'you shouldn't be as sad, you had the chance to see them one last time, come on now . . . get over it!'. Instead of offering up a thought or a statement unprompted, the best thing you can do is lend an ear and hold space for that person.

Here are some phrases to avoid.

- 'They're in a better place.'
- 'They wouldn't want you to be sad.'
- 'Everything happens for a reason.'
- 'It was their time to go.'
- 'They lived a good life.'
- 'It was meant to be.'
- 'You'll find someone else.'

If you read this list and thought, *Argh . . . I've said a few of these things!*, don't stress, you're not the only one. Just remember for next time.

DON'T COMPARE

Whatever you do, however much you want to, don't compare losses. Refrain from saying things like, 'I know how you feel. I lost my dog and . . . ', 'It could be worse' or 'I know someone who . . . '.

This is not the time to share your experiences, or try to compare. The griever is in so much pain and they don't care who has had it worse.

Trying to share your similar experience might seem helpful, but it can come across as dismissive. Our advice? Avoid comparisons at all costs.

TAKE THEIR LEAD WITH THE LANGUAGE YOU USE

Ah, euphemisms! We use indirect language to convey a word that may be considered too blunt – like died, dead, death and dying. Do you dare say it, or do you say 'passed away', 'passed', 'gone', 'lost' or 'passed on'?

You might be scared to say the wrong thing, or seem blunt or rude. To be honest, it is so unique to the individual. Some people hate softening the language by saying 'passed away' or 'lost'. They prefer saying how it is: 'They died.' Other people find this too confronting. It's best to suss it out with the person. Notice what language they use and take their lead.

Respect the boundaries of the person who's grieving. Some people like to talk and let it all out. Other people prefer to process things alone. It's a good idea to ask, 'Would you like to talk about it?' or 'Are you okay if I talk about them?' Ask if they would be comfortable before you broach the subject and, if they say no, then don't go there.

SUPPORT THEM ON DIFFICULT DAYS

It takes less than one minute to make a quick note of the 'big days'. By this, we mean the date the person died, anniversaries, the birthday of the person who died, or the grieving person's birthday. Basically, days when they might be thinking about their person extra hard, or really feeling the loss.

It takes minimal effort to send a text to say, 'I am thinking of you today', but for someone who is grieving, it can make a massive difference. By reaching out, you show them that you remember the person who has died. It shows them that you are there for support, and that you understand it is a tough day for them. It can mean so much to the person grieving to hear from you on that day.

Also, check-in on the non-big days occasionally, too. Sometimes a random Tuesday might feel just as full of grief and hurt as the date that their person died.

BE CONSIDERATE AROUND THE HOLIDAY SEASON

Some people who are grieving can find holidays, such as Christmas, especially difficult. They might struggle to feel celebratory or jolly. If you're spending a holiday with someone who is coping with loss, understand that they might not be feeling super social. Respect their choice if they want to keep things low-key.

On the other hand, some people find holidays lonely and crave company. If you have a spare seat at the table and know someone who is grieving, why not invite them over? Ask them what might feel good for them on the day. If they accept your invitation, try to talk about their person, or raise a glass in their memory.

TIPS FOR MANAGERS AND COLLEAGUES

Our work takes up a huge part of our lives and colleagues can become like friends and family. Supporting an employee or colleague who is grieving is so important. These tips might help.

- **Let them know that their workload is taken care of** and that there's no expectation to check emails.

- **Offer a plan for their return.** It might be flexible working or part-time hours, splitting their workload, regular breaks or organising for them to see a grief counsellor.

- **Take your cues from the griever** before asking them any personal information about their loss. Respect their privacy if they don't want to talk about the loss.

- **It's okay to say their person's name.** If they give you signals that they are comfortable talking about their person, then don't be afraid to say their name or ask a question about them.

- **Be patient.** Remember that grief is ongoing and can flare up months or years later. An employee who came back to work after a few weeks may still need time off later down the line to process their loss.

- **Understand that their work might be inconsistent.** Grief impacts concentration and decision-making, and there can be a lot of brain fog and anxiety that accompanies grief. It can make reading even a simple email feel like a huge task. Communicate clearly that you understand this, and offer support and guidance.

CARING FOR A CARER

When you think of grief, you might think of the grief that comes with losing someone. However, many of our community members have experienced anticipatory grief, which is the grief that comes when you are *anticipating* the loss of someone you love. Someone might be caring for a loved one with a terminal diagnosis, or a family member with dementia. This can be incredibly difficult. Not only are they providing physical and emotional support to the person, but often others, too. They may also be feeling grief for the person in their care, even though they haven't yet died, which can be exhausting, both emotionally and physically.

When someone is a carer, they need to be cared for, too. Offer to take them for a coffee and a chat. Cook them dinner so they can take that off their list for one evening. If you have the spare cash, treat them to a massage. If they have kids, offer to look after them for an hour or two so they can have some time alone.

BE A GRIEF ALLY

Our final tip is this: be a grief advocate. If you have found this chapter helpful, pass this book on to others. Spread the word about how to show up and support those who are grieving. Let others know what grief is like and how it can impact people. Let them know what they can expect, what they can say and not say. Help raise awareness that grief doesn't last only a few months or a year. You can help smash the taboo around this topic. Yes, *you*!

IN TIME, YOUR GRIEF MAY FEEL LESS LIKE

pain

AND MORE LIKE

love.

THANK YOU ...

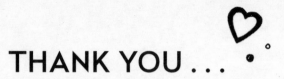

This book was written in honour of our mums, Rose and Vanessa. Without them, Good Mourning would not be. Thank you for the years we had together and for being the inspiration behind everything we do. We hope we are doing you proud.

To Julie Mazur Tribe, Virginia Birch, Sarah Hatton and the team at Murdoch Books, for believing in this book and giving us your full support and guidance throughout. To our editor, Justine Harding, for your care and ability to piece together our puzzles! We are so grateful for your understanding and patience, and for helping us make this book what it is. To our design manager, Sarah Odgers, and our illustrator, Sarah Campbell, for helping us bring our creative design vision to life, and to our designer, Madeleine Kane, for your incredible design skills and for making the book look beautiful. To Tamara Cavenett and the team at the Australian Psychological Association, for sharing your professional insights and coming on this journey with us.

To our other halves, Ant and Ben, for encouraging us to give Good Mourning a go in the first place, and for all the podcast editing, website design, late nights, and steadfast love and support. We owe you a lifetime of Maccas.

To our families and friends, for being light in the dark and for constant support. There are way too many to name here (it would end up being a whole book in itself!), but we love you all, and you know who you are.

To everyone who sent us messages and rallied around us during the hard (and not-so-hard) times.

To Sandra Bridekirk, for giving us your unfiltered feedback and reassurance. We are so grateful for you.

To Andre Sikanjic, for your design skills and always lending a hand, and to Jack Phillips and Mark Sherborne for your photography skills.

To Louisa Smith and the team at Griefline for your support, and to Motherless Daughters Australia for giving us the opportunity to meet.

To all our incredible podcast guests – each and every one of you has made Good Mourning what it is today.

To our Good Mourning listeners and grief community – thank you for being with us every step of the way. We wouldn't be able to do any of this without you.

And lastly, to our community members who so bravely shared your stories for this book. You are all amazing, and we are forever grateful. We hope that you feel your voices are reflected throughout these pages.

RESOURCES

Extra grief support for you, no matter
where you might be on your journey.

Connect with us at @goodmourningpodcast on Instagram or come and say
hello at goodmourning.com.au.

Australia

- **Australian Centre for Grief
  and Bereavement (ACGB)** is
  the largest provider of grief and
  bereavement education in Australia:
  grief.org.au
- **First Light Widowed Association**
  connects young widowed people
  to resources, programs and a
  community that will support them:
  firstlight.org.au
- **Griefline** offers phone counselling
  services, online forums, and tools
  and resources to offer hope and
  healing after loss: **griefline.org.au**

- **Motherless Daughters Australia**
  provides support services to girls
  and women who have experienced
  mother loss: **motherlessdaughters.
  com.au**
- **Pink Elephants** offer resources,
  information and peer support for
  those impacted by early pregnancy
  loss: **pinkelephants.org.au**
- **Wings of Hope** provides resources
  and support for people who are
  bereaved by suicide: **wingsofhope.
  org.au**

United Kingdom

- **Cruse Bereavement Support**
  provides support and information
  on bereavement: **cruse.org.uk**
- **The Good Grief Trust** is a great
  resource for information around
  different grief support throughout
  the UK: **thegoodgrieftrust.org**
- **Marie Curie** provides nursing
  and hospice care, a free support
  line, and information and support
  on all aspects of dying, death and
  bereavement: **mariecurie.org.uk**

- **The New Normal Charity
  (TNN)** offers free peer-to-peer
  grief support groups for people
  coping with grief and loss:
  thenewnormalcharity.com
- **Sibling Grief Club** offers support
  and resources for bereaved adult
  siblings: **siblinggriefclub.com**
- **SUDEP Action** is a UK charity
  specialising in supporting people
  bereaved by epilepsy: **sudep.org**

- **Sue Ryder** is a charity that supports the bereaved and those living with a terminal illness: **sueryder.org**

- **Talk About Loss** runs meet-ups across the UK for bereaved young people: **letstalkaboutloss.org**

United States of America and Canada

- **Alliance of Hope** offers support to those grieving after a suicide: **allianceofhope.org**

- **The Dinner Party** offers peer grief support through regular community events: **thedinnerparty.org**

- **Grief.com** offers grief support through education, information and other helpful resources: **grief.com**

- **Modern Loss** is an excellent website offering candid content, resources and community for loss and grief: **modernloss.com**

- **Refuge in Grief** has a wealth of grief support resources from psychotherapist and author Megan Devine: **refugeingrief.com**

- **What's Your Grief** is an excellent website full of resources related to understanding and coping with grief and loss: **whatsyourgrief.com**

Books

- *The AfterGrief: Finding your way along the long arc of loss* by Hope Edelman (Ballantine Books, 2020)

- *Anxiety: The missing stage of grief: A revolutionary approach to understanding and healing the impact of loss* by Claire Bidwell Smith (Da Capo Lifelong Books, 2018)

- *The Body Keeps the Score: Brain, mind, and body in the healing of trauma* by Bessel van der Kolk (Penguin, 2014)

- *The Choice: A true story of hope* by Edith Eger (Rider – Trade, 2018)

- *Finding Meaning: The sixth stage of grief* by David Kessler (Scribner, 2019)

- *Grief: A guided journal* by Jo Betz (2021)

- *Grief Works: Stories of life, death and surviving* by Julia Samuel (Penguin Life, 2018)

- *The Hot Young Widows Club: Lessons on survival from the front lines of grief* by Nora McInerny (Simon & Schuster/TED, 2019)

- *It's OK That You're Not OK: Meeting grief and loss in a culture that doesn't understand* by Megan Devine (Sounds True, 2017)

- *Signs: The secret language of the universe* by Laura Lynne Jackson (Piaktus, 2019)

- *Surviving Death: A journalist investigates evidence for an afterlife* by Leslie Kean (Crown, 2017)

NOTES

CHAPTER 1: The Elephant in the Room

Kübler-Ross, E., *On Death and Dying*, New York: Scribner, 1997

Zagdanski, D., 'Factsheet 24: Intuitive vs instrumental grievers', *My Grief Assist*, 2014 <mygriefassist.com.au/content/dam/invocare/mygriefassist/factsheets-PDFs/factsheet_24_instrumental_vs_intuitive.pdf>

Keller, S., 'On Grieving Styles', *The Center for Loss and Bereavement*, 16 November 2016 <bereavementcenter.org/on-grieving-styles>

Williams, L., 'Secondary Loss – one loss isn't enough??!!', *What's Your Grief*, 22 July 2013 <whatsyourgrief.com/secondary-loss-one-loss-isnt-enough>

Williams, L., 'How do I know I'm experiencing complicated grief?', *What's Your Grief*, 2012 <whatsyourgrief.com/normal-or-not-so-normal-grief>

Tonkin, L., 'Growing around grief – another way of looking at grief and recovery', *Bereavement Care*, 1 March 1996, vol. 15, no. 1, p. 10 <doi.org/10.1080/02682629608657376>

Edelman, H., *The AfterGrief: Finding your way along the long arc of loss*, New York: Ballentine Books, 2020, pp. 12, 15

CHAPTER 2: Emotional All-sorts

Devine, M., *It's OK That You're Not OK: Meeting grief and loss in a culture that doesn't understand*, Boulder: Sounds True, 2017, pp. 81, 82

Benson, K. 'The Anger Iceberg', *The Gottman Institute*, 8 November 2016 <gottman.com/blog/the-anger-iceberg>

Brown, B., *Daring Greatly: How the courage to be vulnerable transforms the way we live, love, parent, and lead*, London: Penguin, 2013, p. 2

Gračanin, A., Bylsma, L.M. & Vingerhoets, A.J.J.M., 'Is crying a self-soothing behavior?', *Frontiers in Psychology*, 28 May 2014, vol. 5, no. 502 <doi.org/10.3389/fpsyg.2014.00502>

Stroebe, M. & Schut, H., 'The dual process model of coping with bereavement: rationale and description', *Death Studies*, 1999, vol. 23, no. 3, pp.197–224 <doi.org/10.1080/074811899201046>

CHAPTER 3: When Grief Gets Physical

Monk, T.H., Germain, A. & Reynolds, C.F., 'Sleep Disturbance in Bereavement', *Psychiatric Annals*, 1 October 2008, vol. 38, no. 10, pp. 671–75 <doi.org/10.3928/00485713-20081001-06>

Shulman, L.M., 'Healing the Brain After Loss': Webinar, American Brain Foundation, 25 June 2021 <youtu.be/hZwhslOz7qY>

Sarner, M., 'Brain fog: how trauma, uncertainty and isolation have affected our minds and memory', *The Guardian*, 14 April 2021 <theguardian.com/lifeandstyle/2021/apr/14/brain-fog-how-trauma-uncertainty-and-isolation-have-affected-our-minds-and-memory>

Division of Sleep Medicine at Harvard Medical School, 'Sleep, Learning and Memory', *Healthy Sleep*, 18 December 2007 <healthysleep.med.harvard.edu/healthy/matters/benefits-of-sleep/learning-memory>

Smith, C.B., *Anxiety: The missing stage of grief: A revolutionary approach to understanding and healing the impact of loss*, Boston: Da Capo Lifelong Books, 2018, pp. 19, 21, 33

Van der Kolk, B., *The Body Keeps the Score: Brain, mind, and body in the healing of trauma*, New York: Penguin, 2014, pp. 53–4

Seliger, I., 'The Biology of Grief', *The New York Times*, 22 April 2021 <nytimes.com/2021/04/22/well/what-happens-in-the-body-during-grief.html>

CHAPTER 4: Self-care for Grievers

APA Dictionary of Psychology, 'burnout', *American Psychological Association*, 2022 <dictionary.apa.org/burnout>

Tawwab, N.G., *Set Boundaries, Find Peace: A guide to reclaiming yourself*, London: Piatkus, 2021, p. 4

'Self-care interventions for health', *World Health Organization* (WHO), 30 June 2022, <who.int/news-room/fact-sheets/detail/self-care-health-interventions>

CHAPTER 5: You, Me and Grief

Devine, M., 'Grief changes your address book . . . ', on Twitter @refugeingrief, 14 June 2021 <twitter.com/refugeingrief/status/1404423430175404035>

'DEAR MAN Skill', *DBT Tools*, 2022 <dbt.tools/interpersonal_effectiveness/dear-man.php>

Devine, M., 'The hierarchy of grief: Some people are at the periphery', *Refuge in Grief*, 14 August 2017 <refugeingrief.com/2017/08/14/hierarchy>

Devine, M., *It's OK That You're Not OK: Meeting grief and loss in a culture that doesn't understand*, Boulder: Sounds True, 2017, p. 17

CHAPTER 6: You Are Not Alone

Haley, E., 'The Unique Loneliness of Grief', *What's Your Grief*, 2 August 2016 <whatsyourgrief.com/unique-loneliness-grief>

Jennings-Edquist, G., 'What it's like to be a young widow', *ABC Everyday*, 29 June 2021 <abc.net.au/everyday/what-it-is-like-to-be-a-young-widow/100252118#:~:text=As%20a%20young%20person%2C%20grieving,grief%20expert%20Dr%20Lauren%20Breen>

Marshall, C., 'How to Overcome Loneliness', *Self Space*, 2020 <theselfspace.com/overcoming-loneliness>

CHAPTER 8: Gone, But Not Forgotten

Klass, D., Silverman, P.R. & Nickman S.L. (eds.), *Continuing Bonds: New understandings of grief*, Washington, DC: Taylor and Francis, 1996

Jackson, L.L., *Signs: The secret language of the universe*, London: Piatkus, 2019, pp. xvi, xvii, 156, 157

CONCLUSION

McInerny, N., 'We don't "move on" from grief. We move forward with it', TEDwomen, November 2018 <ted.com/talks/nora_mcinerny_we_don_t_move_on_from_grief_we_move_forward_with_it>

INDEX

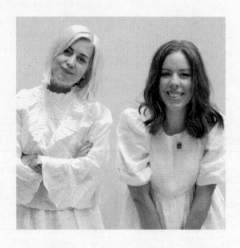

Sally Douglas and Imogen Carn
are co-hosts of the top-rated
podcast Good Mourning and
creators of the Instagram account
@goodmourningpodcast.